PERFECT SKIN

PERFECT SKIN

JANET FILDERMAN

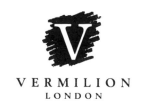

VERMILION
LONDON

DEDICATION

I would like to dedicate this book to my many clients who, by their loyalty, love and interest, have been so inspirational.

Published in 1992 by Vermilion
an imprint of Ebury Press
Random Century House
20 Vauxhall Bridge Road
London SW1V 2SA

British Library Cataloguing-in-Publication Data
Filderman, Janet
Perfect skin.
I. Title
646.7

ISBN 0-09-175177-2

Editor: Alison Wormleighton
Designers: Janet James and Jerry Goldie
Photographer: Jon Stewart
Illustrator: Mike Breese
Photograph on page 9 by John Deehan

Typeset in Futura by Textype Typesetters, Cambridge
Printed and bound in Great Britain by
Butler and Tanner Ltd., Frome and London

CONTENTS

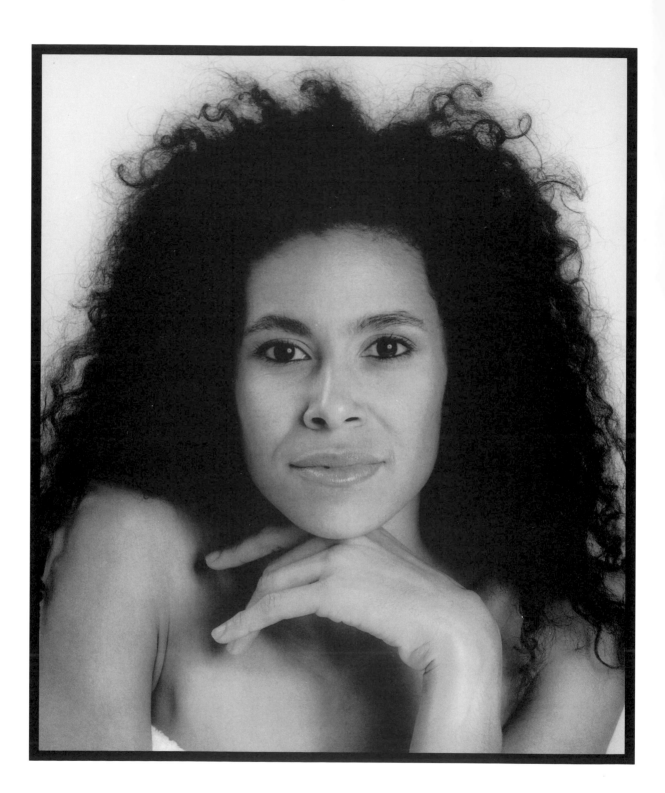

FOREWORD

Janet Filderman has, above all, been my friend for many years; I know of few people who could combine such great skill with the added bonus of being such a smashing person to be with.

Her professionalism, wealth of knowledge and sheer charm are legendary. The skin products she has formulated and developed personally are in testimony to her practical, no-nonsense approach to skin care, as are the results.

Janet is my choice for the best in her business and I hope that this book will give many readers a real insight into her remarkable talent and wonderful personality.

Barbara

Barbara Daly

INTRODUCTION

I have always been interested in beauty and began to take care of my skin from early adolescence. From trial and error, I found out that because my skin was oily I was constantly being sold beauty products which were too astringent, resulting in dry patches and irritations. So I began to treat my skin as I thought it should be treated — very gently. I used products for sensitive skin and it began to work. The oily centre panel started to behave better and gave little trouble because I was not over-stimulating it. I was spot-free.

In my early twenties I secured a position as private secretary to a cancer surgeon. It was while in this job that I began to take an interest in how the body works. The surgeon encouraged me to ask questions and I became fascinated by the skin and how it functions. I was allowed to help by preparing the trolley with sterilized instruments and to assist in minor surgical procedures. It was this surgeon's suggestion that I would make a good beauty therapist which eventually galvanized me to take a beauty therapy course when I moved from my Yorkshire home to London.

I took a course with the Innoxa Beauty School in the early 1960s and worked for this excellent company for the next five years. Their products were hypo-allergenic and unperfumed long before it became fashionable. I am sure that my time with them was the best foundation I could have had.

My career in beauty was further advanced when I was approached by Christian Dior, just before they launched their skin care range, to teach product knowledge to beauty consultants. This was followed

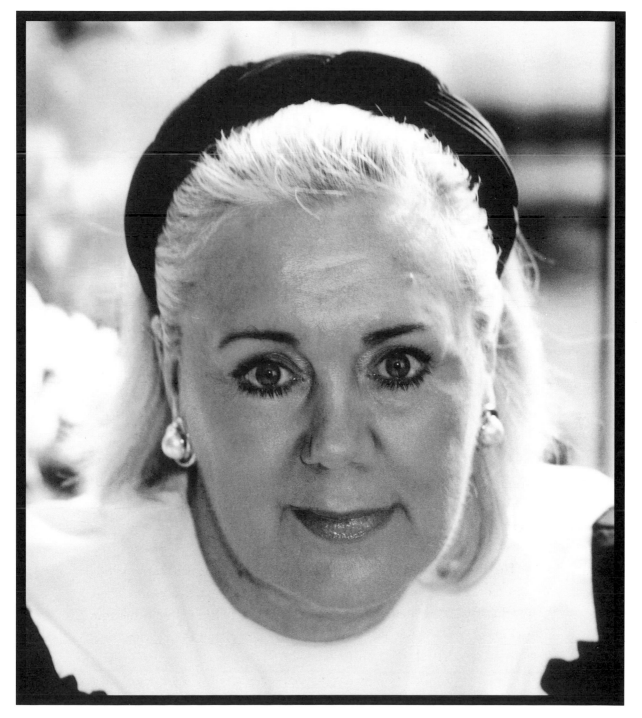

Janet Filderman

by three years at Charles of the Ritz training their consultants. It was a stimulating and interesting job though it required a great deal of time travelling the country.

These positions enabled me to see the beauty industry from the sales and marketing side, but my greatest treat was the opportunity to discuss the reasons for the development of new creams with the cosmetic chemists.

I had been in the beauty business for about fifteen years when, feeling a little depressed by the marketing hype, I was encouraged by a

' A beautician has a unique and special relationship with her client. '

friend – Dr Tom Elliot, a cosmetic chemist of brilliance and great panache – to set up my own salon. I have loved every minute of it, yet it has never been my wish to have a chain of salons. I feel that the beautician has a unique and special relationship with her client which cannot be passed on without it getting 'watered down'. Each operator has her own way of linking with her client, and when one is so close, vulnerability and sensitivity are important factors. A mutual liking and respect have to be established for the relationship to last and be of benefit.

I am deeply interested in how the body works and how the skin responds to the elements and general wear-and-tear of the passing years, and I try to help and advise my clients and mail order customers, to avoid the hype of the beauty industry.

It is not the job of the beauticians and beauty houses to promote the Dorian Gray principle. Their job should be to encourage the care of skin – not to give the impression that eternal youth can be obtained from a jar of cream or a special salon treatment. Creating false hopes only leads to unhappiness because the customer then believes that she has failed. She sees the years leaving their mark and her efforts seem wasted.

When I was approached to write this book on beauty, I had a definite view on what I wanted to aim for – a positive approach with no drivel. There would be no claims of miracles, no suggestion of rejuvenating creams to create a younger-looking you. Instead, the purpose of this book is to show you how to achieve your own particular beauty, based on health and vitality and soft, glowing skin. This book will enable you to give yourself a complete beauty make-over, transforming your image from top to toe. I am obviously not suggesting you will become another Joan Collins or Jane Fonda. My objective is to give you professional advice which is normally only available to the privileged few. I want to make you aware of your own style and potential.

Most women lack self-confidence – which is why we have role models. We are always wishing we were like, say, the Princess of Wales, or Elizabeth Taylor. (You never hear men wishing they were Clint Eastwood or Chris de Burgh. They do not bother too much if they are bald and out of condition. That's self-confidence!) Admiring

> **6** *My objective is to give you professional advice which is normally only available to the privileged few.* **9**

someone for their achievements in life is a normal reaction; the danger lies in becoming depressed with our lives because we cannot be like them.

We must each find our own key and develop ourselves. That is the secret our role models have found: having developed their own potential, they project it so that it becomes their trademark. It does not come easily and it requires a great deal of self-discipline, but the rewards are extremely fulfilling.

This is your opportunity to gain the confidence and ability to allow your own individual style, your particular beauty, to develop fully. And beauty begins with a radiant complexion.

CHAPTER ONE

UNDERSTANDING YOUR SKIN

S kin is the largest organ of the body and, apart from the brain, the most complex one. It is not given much attention until it goes wrong, and it is very misunderstood. If you wish to have a glowing complexion, then you must learn to understand it and allow it to function in the way nature intended. All those articles that appear in magazines suggesting that if you use this or that cream you will have no wrinkles or will rejuvenate your skin fail to take into account that skin is a living part of you.

It is my intention to guide you towards greater knowledge of how your skin works and how it reacts to everyday living, thus preventing you from ever again feeling confused or uncertain when confronted with the vast array of beauty products on the cosmetic counters.

THE FUNCTION OF SKIN

Skin is your protection against the world. The outermost covering of the body, it protects your internal organs from damage and the environment. Skin acts as a two-way barrier, preventing loss of water, electrolytes and fluids from the body, and barring the entry of harmful substances. In addition, it is a sensory organ, containing over five billion sensory nerve cells and transmitting to the brain signals such as itching, pain, heat or cold. It controls body temperature, dilating tiny blood vessels in the skin when signalled by the brain to do so, and it gets rid of waste matter. If you are ill or tired, your skin will quickly show it.

The skin contains a fatty substance to make it waterproof – your own natural moisturizer. Its unique water-retaining capacity contributes to its elasticity and helps to maintain the body's balance of fluids. (Young skin actually contains about 8 litres/14 pints of water, which is the main reason for its plumpness.)

The skin consists of two layers: a thin outer layer, the epidermis, and a thicker, inner layer, the dermis. Beneath the dermis is the subcutaneous fat layer, which gives the skin its cushion and helps to shield the vital organs.

The outermost layer, the epidermis, is made up of flat, dead cells.

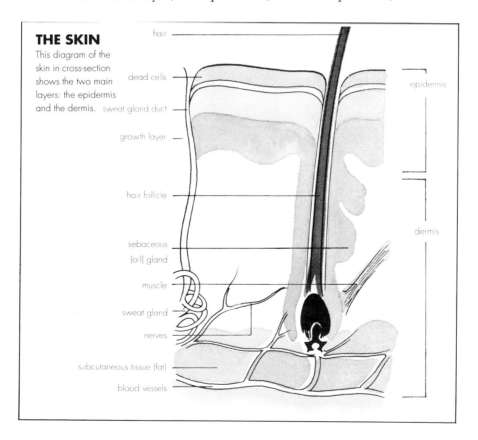

THE SKIN

This diagram of the skin in cross-section shows the two main layers: the epidermis and the dermis.

hair

dead cells

sweat gland duct

growth layer

hair follicle

sebaceous (oil) gland

muscle

sweat gland

nerves

subcutaneous tissue (fat)

blood vessels

epidermis

dermis

About the thickness of clingfilm, it is slightly thicker on the palms of the hands and soles of the feet and is thinner around the eyes. Normally, men have a thicker epidermis than women, but it usually thins down in both sexes with age. As the epidermal cells wear away, they are replaced by living cells from the lower part of the epidermis, known as the basal cell layer. One of the functions of this layer of cells is to produce a substance called keratin, which is a hard protein. Hair and nails are extensions of the skin and are mainly composed of keratin. Melanin is also produced in this layer, giving the skin its colour (more about this on page 103).

The dermis is sometimes called the 'true skin', for it consists of living cells interspersed with connective tissue, blood vessels, hair follicles, sweat glands and sebaceous glands, the openings of which are the pores on the surface of the skin.

The sebaceous glands produce an oily substance which mixes with the sweat and becomes the body's natural moisturizer when it reaches

> **6 *With gentle handling, the skin's surface can be greatly improved. But be suspicious of any products that claim to penetrate deep into the skin.* 9**

the outer layer of the skin. Sebaceous glands are not distributed evenly all over the body but are concentrated in particular areas. For instance, there is a high concentration of them around the nose but very few under the eyes.

Wrinkles and cellular renewal

The beauty business is only concerned with the epidermis – which, with gentle handling, can be greatly improved. The thousands of microscopic lines on the skin's surface can be smoothed out, so that the skin reflects light better and looks firmer. Yet it is the condition of the underlying connective tissues in the dermis which determines the extent of a person's lines and wrinkles. In young skin, the collagen and elastin fibres present in these tissues provide firm, springy support for the epidermis. As skin ages, the support gradually deteriorates, rather like an old mattress.

The dermis cannot be reached externally by any cosmetic product or by a beautician, despite the implications to the contrary of some cosmetic manufacturers. Products that can penetrate to the dermis are classified not as cosmetics but as drugs. Recently, there has been a great scientific interest in cellular renewal. Scientists have managed to reprogramme DNA, the genetic blueprint of cells. It is a most exciting field and will probably be used first to treat cancers; however, a great deal of research is still needed. Any claim that a cosmetic product can affect cellular renewal should be regarded with a great deal of suspicion and could do an enormous amount of damage in the hands of non-medical personnel.

BEAUTY FROM WITHIN

The cells in the skin are continually renewing themselves. To give them a good start in life, you need to have a proper diet and a healthy lifestyle, with plenty of fresh air, exercise and sleep.

Diet

Aim for a balanced diet rich in fresh fruits and vegetables, especially leafy green vegetables, and wholemeal bread, rice, pasta and cereal. Make sure your protein intake includes a reasonable proportion of fish and chicken, and also pulses, but not too much red meat. Low-fat dairy products are important too. Aim to keep your sugar and fat consumption low (though you musn't eliminate fat entirely) and avoid processed foods. This is a recipe for a healthy body in general, and it will show itself in your skin, hair and nails, as well as your overall energy level.

I am a big believer in vitamin and mineral supplements. But even if you choose not to use supplements, it is important to be aware of your vitamin and mineral intake. Also, remember that the body can store some vitamins (A, D, E and K) but not the vitamins in the B complex or vitamin C, and minerals are not easily stored, so you need to make sure you are getting a daily intake of these.

Alcohol

Alcohol depletes the body of amino acids and slows down cellular renewal. (In fact, heavy drinking robs the body of virtually every vital nutrient and causes tissues to retain body fluids, as well as being responsible for damage to the brain and liver.) Alcohol also makes the skin drier and causes tiny blood vessels in the face to dilate, promoting capillary damage.

Smoking

Apart from its effects on health, smoking reduces the amount of oxygen that gets to the skin, which affects collagen fibres, and it depletes the body of vitamin C. It also dries out and yellows the skin and leads to premature lines around the eyes and mouth.

Lifestyle

The way you live will show in your face. Too much stress aggravates many skin conditions (see pages 35, 36, 37 and 88-9). Exercise, on the other hand, not only makes you feel better and more energetic, but it also boosts your metabolism and your circulation, thereby perking up the complexion. Some studies suggest that regular, vigorous exercise also speeds up cell renewal and slows down the skin's ageing process.

Enough sleep is essential too (though requirements vary from person to person). Between midnight and 4am is when the skin cells work overtime to repair and renew themselves. Lack of sleep results in grey-looking, puffy skin with a poor texture.

QUESTIONS FROM CLIENTS

Is skin really thicker in some places than others?

The soles of the feet and the palms of the hands are areas of
the body that produce a thicker surface than, say, on the face
or body – this is quite understandable when you think of
the tremendous amount of use these areas get. We walk
many miles during our normal lifetime and the feet take a
great deal of pounding. Professional walkers even prepare
their feet by using spirit to harden the sole and to prevent
blisters forming when walking or running marathons.
Manual workers develop callouses on the palms which
reinforce the epidermis to prevent damage to the inner skin.
Some musicians also develop callouses from playing
particular instruments. It is important to keep these thicker
areas in good order by massaging regularly with body
creams or lotions.

Do I need a vitamin supplement?

If you live in a town and have to buy food from a
supermarket, if you are stressed, if you are recovering from
an illness, or if for some reason you are unable to obtain a
good range of whole, fresh food (see page 15), I would most
certainly recommend a multi-vitamin and mineral
supplement. You do not have to go mad and overdo things
but I am sure you would notice the difference. If you have
itchy skin, cracked lips or splitting nails, these can be
helped with a vitamin supplement.
If you are pregnant or if you are taking any form of drugs
prescribed by your doctor, you should discuss the question
with him before undertaking any other forms of treatment.

CHAPTER TWO

DAY-TO-DAY COMPLEXION CARE

The beauty industry has a vested interest in promoting more and more exaggerated claims for cosmetics, and persuading women to use as many different products in a day as possible. But I am convinced that more than 90 per cent of skin troubles are caused by over-use of products.

Women have been brainwashed into thinking that by using more skin-care cosmetics they will slow down the onset of ageing of the skin, but, in fact, this can lead to congested pores and the suppression of the skin's own natural protection.

LESS IS BEST

My philosophy is simple and is based on the fact that less is best. It involves getting back to basics and letting the skin look after itself. Good skin relies on healthy cellular renewal, not on some miraculous wonder cream.

The plethora of facial creams and gels, scrubs and lotions is very bewildering for anyone not in the beauty business. However, there are only a few products that you actually need: a cleanser, perhaps a toner, a moisturizer and possibly a conditioning cream. The skin care routines which I recommend in this book have worked for my clients

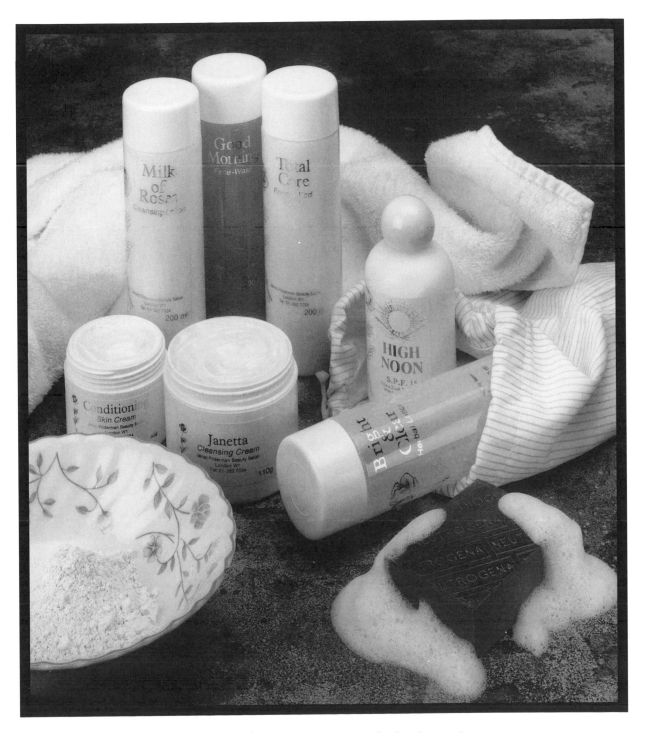

To look after your skin properly you need only a few products.

and they will work for you. It doesn't matter whether your skin tone is pale and translucent, fair and freckled, medium-toned, olive or dark – these regimes will improve your skin.

Cleansing cream or lotion

The main function of a cleansing cream or lotion is to clean make-up and day-to-day grime from the skin without stripping away all the skin's natural oils. An effective cleanser, therefore, must have the right proportions of oily and non-oily ingredients, in order to achieve

More than 90 per cent of skin troubles are caused by over-use of beauty products. Women have been brainwashed into thinking that they need them all.

a perfect balance between cleansing and conditioning. Creams are richer (ie, oilier) than lotions and consequently suitable for drier complexions. Some cleansers, known as facial washes, are lathered up like soap with water and then rinsed off with water; these will not remove make-up successfully because the molecules are too large to penetrate the skin, so surface cleaning is their main function.

Normal soaps are too alkaline and tend to dry out the surface of the skin. Furthermore, they do not penetrate the epidermis and therefore are not satisfactory as a cleaning agent if make-up is worn. Instead, look for non-alkaline soaps such as transparent glycerine bars. 'Cleansing bars' are cleansers in solid form which have a lathering agent added to give the appearance of soap.

Toner

The main purpose of a toning product originally was to remove any remaining traces of cleanser, but cleansers are no longer as heavy as they once were, so water can be used instead of toner and is less drying to the skin. However, toners do make the skin feel fresh and tingly, and some women like to use one after cleansing. (It should not be used instead of cleanser.)

Traditionally, fresheners and tonics have been the mildest of the toning products, followed by toners, with astringents the strongest. Astringents contain alcohol, supposedly to 'close' the pores of oily skin. But pores are not like shutters that can be opened and closed, and the effect is actually created by the alcohol causing the capillaries to dilate and the tiny erectile muscles of the pores to tighten, making

> *You actually need only a few products to look after your skin: a cleanser, a moisturizer and, if your skin is dry, a conditioning cream.*

the pores look smaller temporarily. Alcohol, is, however, too harsh even for the oiliest skin, and these days toning products more often contain various plant extracts such as witch hazel, menthol or camphor. Nevertheless, all toning products should be used with care, as they can be drying when used daily. They should be avoided entirely if the skin is damaged.

Moisturizer

The purpose of moisturizing lotions and creams is not to add moisture but to aid moisture retention. In other words, a moisturizer provides a waterproof 'raincoat' for the skin preventing premature moisture loss. A moisturizer also softens the skin, making it smoother and more supple. As with cleansers, a cream is richer than a lotion and therefore suitable for drier complexions.

In an effort to stand out from the crowd, many moisturizers contain a variety of special ingredients which are supposed to bring added benefits, ranging from increasing the skin's oxygen supply to encouraging cell renewal. However, these added benefits (for which you pay a considerable price) are, at best, marginal.

Conditioning creams – often called 'nourishing creams' – are lubricating creams which contain a much higher proportion of oil than moisturizing lotions do. Whereas the high water content of moisturizers prevents them from penetrating into the skin, the low water content of conditioning creams relative to the high proportion of oil allows them to penetrate very slightly into the top layer of the skin to lubricate it effectively.

Conditioning creams are often called 'night creams' because it is sometimes suggested they be used at night (when you don't mind wearing a relatively oily cream). But I have found that complexions benefit from not using *any* cream at night, thereby allowing skin to function as efficiently as possible. If it *is* applied at bedtime, it should be blotted off after ten minutes.

> 6 *Your complexion will benefit by* **not** *using a night cream, thereby allowing your skin to function as nature intended. Special eye creams and neck creams are completely unnecessary.* 9

Other creams you may come across are eye creams and neck creams. The philosophy behind them is that the skin in these areas is different and so requires a different cream. But this is not so. They will do you no harm, but they are unnecessary, as a good moisturizer or conditioning cream can be used everywhere.

Face mask

The main ingredient of most face masks is one of the natural clays or earths, which can be mixed with water or rosewater to produce a smooth paste that is easy to apply. Therapeutic ingredients such as sulphur or an antiseptic are often added. The purpose of these masks is to extract impurities from the skin; the clay absorbs them so that they are easily washed away. I recommend a kaolin mask (see page 45), which can be made at home very inexpensively, and is extremely effective without drying out the skin.

Clay masks are often described as 'deep-cleansing' products. Two other types of product that are also included in the deep-cleansing

> **6** *Exfoliation is far too harsh for skin,*
> *exposing new cells prematurely.* **9**

category are scrubbing products and chemical peeling products. These, however, do not extract impurities so much as thinning out the dead surface cells (a process known as exfoliation). Scrubbing products – such as scrub creams, cleansing grains, buffing sponges and complexion brushes – literally scrub off the surface debris. Chemical peeling products, also known as clarifying lotions, dissolve some of the cells. My own feeling is that exfoliation is far too harsh for skin, removing cells before they are ready and exposing new cells prematurely. Once again, it is best to allow nature to take its own course at its own pace.

DEFINING YOUR SKIN AND ITS NEEDS

How you use the foregoing products is as important as *what* you use. But before I can recommend a particular regime for you, you need to decide what your skin type is. This is more of a vexed question than people realize. For example, in my many years in the beauty field, I have often been informed by someone that they have a sensitive skin, as though it were a badge of honour. In fact, after a little prodding I usually find that the person has been promoting the condition by overuse of harsh and abrasive products.

The major oil and sweat glands in the face are in what is known as the 'T-panel', which is across the forehead, nose, inner cheeks and chin. When the T-panel gets overworked, by too much use of either drying *or* moisturizing products, congestion of the pores, keratinization (thickening and hardening of the outer cells), dullness and blotchiness occur.

To understand any skin's characteristics and needs, you must first categorize it by age – children's (babyhood to adolescence); adolescent; adult (20 – 50); or mature (50 plus). These categories are then broken down into sensitive, dry, normal, combination and greasy skin, and skin with acne.

Sensitive skin

Sensitive skin can occur at any age and is recognized by a blotchy irritation which can become severe when using perfumed or highly complicated skin care products. It has a tendency to erupt into weals and blisters under the skin; these can begin in the corner of the eyes or eyelids or around the nose. Contrary to popular opinion, this skin

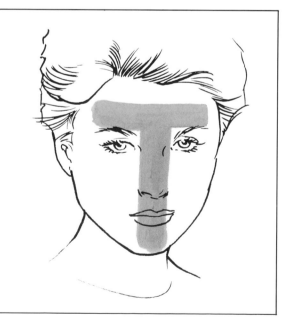

THE T-PANEL

The T-panel – the area across the forehead and down the centre of the face – is where the oil and sweat glands of the face are concentrated. This area does not need moisturizing unless you are elderly or have been ill. In fact, it is the overuse of moisturizers on the T-panel that can lead to many skin problems. The skin must be allowed to function as nature intended – which means that products that dry the skin should not be used either.

can cover all types, from dry to greasy. The calming of the skin should be the first objective before trying to regulate the skin's dryness or oiliness. When the irritations have been calmed and the sensitivity eliminated, then you can begin the slow, gentle routines towards regulating the skin.

Dry skin

Dry skin is apparent when the centre zone of the face does not respond adequately to the demands of the environment and fails to provide the necessary amount of oil and sweat to keep the skin soft and healthy. It has a flaky and tight feel and can also show signs of capillary damage. Creams just 'disappear' into the skin tissue, and a great deal of gentle care is necessary simply to keep it in reasonable order. Dry skin in later age is a normal occurrence, but in a younger person it is important to try to identify the cause and correct it, in order to prevent premature ageing of the skin.

Normal skin

This skin behaves well, with the right amount of oil and sweat being discharged. It has a good, clear texture and colour and the pores are small. This type of skin requires minimal attention, but thorough cleaning is still important, in order to prevent early ageing and clogging effects.

Combination skin

The 'T' panel of combination skin is over-active, resulting in excessive amounts of oil which can lead to blocked pores and an unrefined texture. The outer area of the face can be dry and tight or can behave as normal skin. This is not a difficult skin to deal with if handled correctly. The main problems arise from treating the centre area too harshly. You must treat this type of skin as a normal skin in order to allow the oil glands to slow down; over-stimulation will exacerbate the condition.

Greasy skin

Greasy skin is easier to recognize, because it looks oily and heavy. Open pores and blackheads can be seen down the centre of the face. It can also be accompanied by a slight dryness on the outer part of the face, but you should regard the skin as an oily one and follow the advice given for this type.

Acne

Skin with acne is instantly recognizable by the amount of pustules and blackheads that cover the whole face. If neglected it can be badly scarred and very difficult to correct.

CHILDHOOD

Although most babies are born with perfect skin – not too moist and not too dry – there are some that suffer from atopic eczema. This is an itchy and scaly condition which can be dry or weepy. In small babies it may be associated with asthma. Fortunately, this type of eczema often improves by adolescence.

We take care of babies' skin with tender, gentle routines, scrupulously using baby products rather than harsh soaps. How sad, therefore, that when a child reaches two or three the routine is changed to

*6 Most babies are born with perfect skin.
But often, by the time a child reaches
adolescence, the skin is showing signs of
blocked pores and dry red cheeks. 9*

include ordinary alkali soaps which dry out the skin. Often, by the time the child reaches adolescence the skin is already showing signs of blocked pores and dry red cheeks, or surface dryness, which is then aggravated by the sebaceous glands.

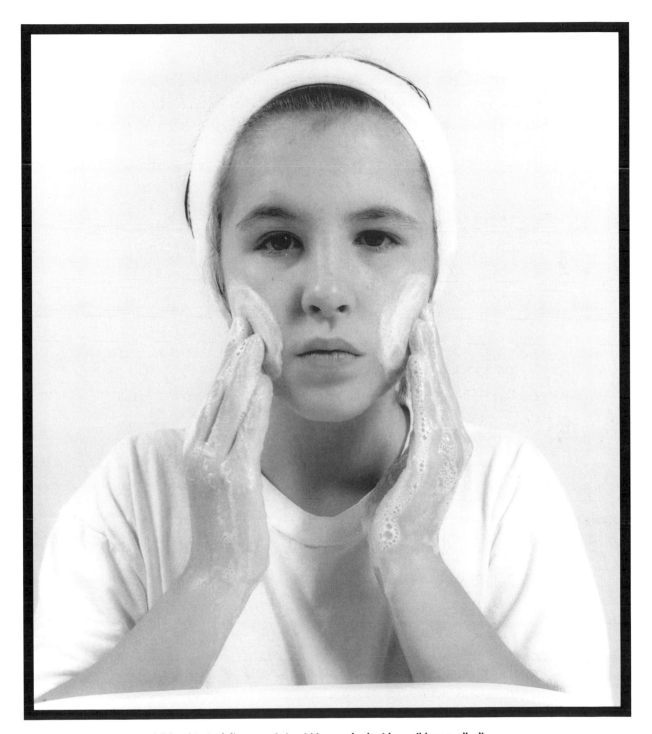

A child's skin is delicate and should be washed with a mild, non-alkali soap.

A child's skin should be cared for by regular washing with a glycerine soap or other mild, non-alkali soap, then rinsed well and carefully patted (not rubbed) dry. Sun protection is absolutely vital (see page 107), as children's skin is very fine and therefore more easily damaged. Body lotion should be used on arms and legs after bathing. School children should be encouraged to look after their skin: a little more care and attention at this stage will reap rewards later in life.

THE TEENAGE YEARS

Adolescence is an exciting but difficult time, often made even more difficult by hormonal changes, which make blocked pores, excessive oiliness and acne the order of the day.

Teenage skin: acne

Acne is a very distressing skin problem for both sexes. Normally, the first sign of impending acne is when blocked pores begin to be infected. It is triggered off by hormonal disturbance, which changes

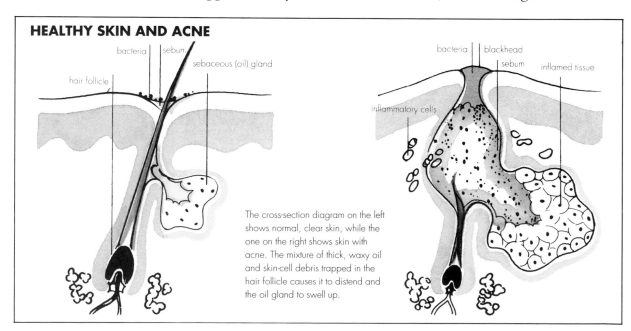

HEALTHY SKIN AND ACNE

bacteria | sebum

sebaceous (oil) gland

hair follicle

bacteria | blackhead

sebum

inflamed tissue

inflammatory cells

The cross-section diagram on the left shows normal, clear skin, while the one on the right shows skin with acne. The mixture of thick, waxy oil and skin-cell debris trapped in the hair follicle causes it to distend and the oil gland to swell up.

the texture of the oil to a waxy substance that is too thick to escape from the pores easily. Then bacteria invades the pores because the body's natural defence mechanism is not working properly. The oiliness is quite different from that of a greasy skin and usually has a stale smell, which is more noticeable on the scalp and back.

Help from a doctor will almost certainly be required in cases of moderate or severe acne. Many doctors advocate antibiotics for this condition because the drug has the advantage of treating the acne from within. It kills the invading bacteria, and at the same time it slows down the oil glands, preventing blockages from occurring. Alternatively, a doctor may prescribe Retin-A, a synthetic derivative of vitamin A. Retin-A is also used to treat sun-damaged skin (see page 91–2).

A doctor would not give a hormone drug to an adolescent because it is assumed that their own hormones will settle down as they advance into their twenties. Acne can, however, develop in later life, and then hormone balancing can be a possible treatment.

To care for skin with acne, you must avoid drying out the outer layer of skin. Cleanse with a mild facial wash and use a topical gel on the pustules if your doctor advises it. Keep the skin clean and free of creams. Never use face masks, scrubs or moisturizers, and do not

> ❛ *With acne, the less that is done to the skin, other than cleansing, the better.* ❜

shave over pustules or raised red lumps. The less that is done to the skin, other than cleaning, the better. Never be tempted to squeeze the blockages – if you do, you will damage the skin and could cause scarring and pitting.

If you possibly can, try to have a monthly facial with a good beautician. In a beautician's hands, the acne client will receive treatment which allows the outer cells to be shed and the oil to flow more freely. A vacuum suction treatment is given which acts like a vacuum

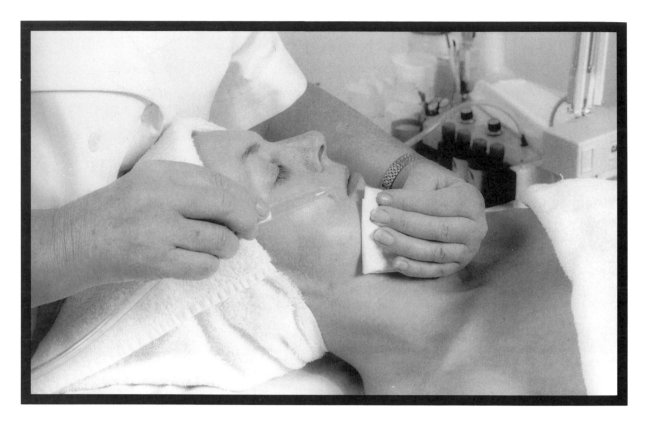

A professional vacuum suction treatment cleans out blocked pores.

cleaner to suck out the blocked sebum from the pores; it does not damage the skin but it can be painful.

If you cannot visit a beautician, you should set about giving yourself a monthly treatment at home. You will need a blackhead extractor (see pages 32 and 48) to dislodge the plug of stale oil that has blocked up the pore. Get one with a dish shape so that you can move it over the nose and chin and the oil will gather in the dish. You use it by placing the hole in the extractor over the blackhead and pressing downwards. The stale oil plug will pop out of the hole and you sterilize the skin with surgical spirit then move on to the next.

If you have acne on your back, it needs to be dealt with in a similar manner, and this is where you must either see a beautician or get a good friend to help you. You need to cleanse the area gently first with a cleansing lotion, then steam the skin (see pages 45 and 47) and finally, with a tissue and an extractor, work gradually over the back to remove the blackheads. Whatever you do, do not touch pustules or raised red lumps. Also, try to wear a clean cotton tee-shirt under day clothes, to prevent bacteria from invading the skin. You could wear one to sleep in, too, but make sure it is clean, since the body releases more oil when you sleep because of the warmth, and a used tee-shirt would spread bacteria.

As a teenager, you may be rushing around missing meals. I would therefore suggest that you take a vitamin/mineral supplement which is designed especially for teenage skin and contains zinc and vitamin Bs. If you are having a course of antibiotics, a daily yogurt (the type containing a live culture) will help restore the bacteria which live in the intestines and are destroyed by antibiotics; the body needs these bacteria for healthy elimination of waste matter.

Teenage skin: greasy

Many teenagers suffer from greasy skin, and it is important they they understand this condition so that they can treat it correctly. A greasy condition can lead to open pores, congestion and dullness. Products which dry the outer layer should never, never be used – they only make the glands produce more oil to compensate. Remember, the

> *Products which dry the outer layer should never, never be used on greasy skin – they only make the glands produce more oils to compensate. Do not use any product which is labelled "for oily skin".*

skin is a living organ and the sensory nerves will react to help you when, in fact, you wanted the opposite. If you keep the skin 'quiet', the message will be a calming one.

If you do not wear make-up, keep the skin clean with a facial wash. If you do wear make-up, cleanse the skin first with a cleansing lotion and then use a facial wash to remove every trace of oil left behind by the cleanser.

Greasy teenage skin does not need a moisturizer. Certainly you should not use one on the T-panel. Moisturizers are sealers and do not allow oil and sweat to escape. Do not use any product which is designated for 'oily' skin or 'acne' – these normally contain drying agents, and an oily skin will react to them by increasing keratinization (hardening and thickening of epidermal cells), which in turn results in congested pores.

This type of skin is prone to spot break-outs, and it is imperative that you do not squeeze them. Squeezing damages the skin by breaking the tiny capillaries and twisting the pore, which prevents new oil from escaping. You could be left with lumps or even permanent marks. When you squeeze, you are in fact increasing the problem by pushing bacteria and pigmented cells into the dermis.

Teenagers with greasy skin often have oily, lank hair and a flaky scalp. If your scalp is flaky, try a medicated dandruff shampoo –

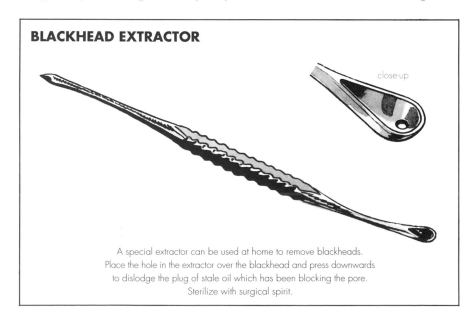

BLACKHEAD EXTRACTOR

close-up

A special extractor can be used at home to remove blackheads.
Place the hole in the extractor over the blackhead and press downwards
to dislodge the plug of stale oil which has been blocking the pore.
Sterilize with surgical spirit.

these are widely available and really do work. You must wash your hair frequently to remove the stale oil and flakes because these flakes tend to stick or fall on to the forehead, where they can cause bacterial infections.

Teenage skin: normal

Normal teenage skin looks like a peach. It has the moistness and colour clarity of glowing good health. The pores are minimal and the sweat and sebaceous glands are functioning without problems. No bacteria enter the skin to cause infection because the skin's natural defence mechanism is working properly. This skin is a joy and is what we all regard as perfect skin.

This is the time when young people are bombarded with media hype to try out the many different skin-care routines and aftershaves. Unfortunately, the tendency is to overuse them, which can have disastrous results because the skin's sensory system will receive the wrong messages.

The daily routine for girls should be simple and, provided cleansing is done carefully, should not take longer than five minutes. It is at

> ❛ *Normal teenage skin looks like a peach.*
> *This skin is a joy and is what we all regard*
> *as perfect skin.* ❜

about this time that girls start to experiment with make-up and it is important that colour pigments are removed from the skin. This can only be done with a cleanser. Oil in the cleanser breaks down sebum and grime on the skin and, at the same time, travels a little way into the skin to lift out the colour pigment that may have penetrated the skin's surface. Cleansing should be done at least twice a day, in the morning and at night. It is essential that make-up is removed thoroughly before going to bed. A night cream is not necessary. In fact, it is better to retire to bed with a clean, fresh skin. A light moisturizing

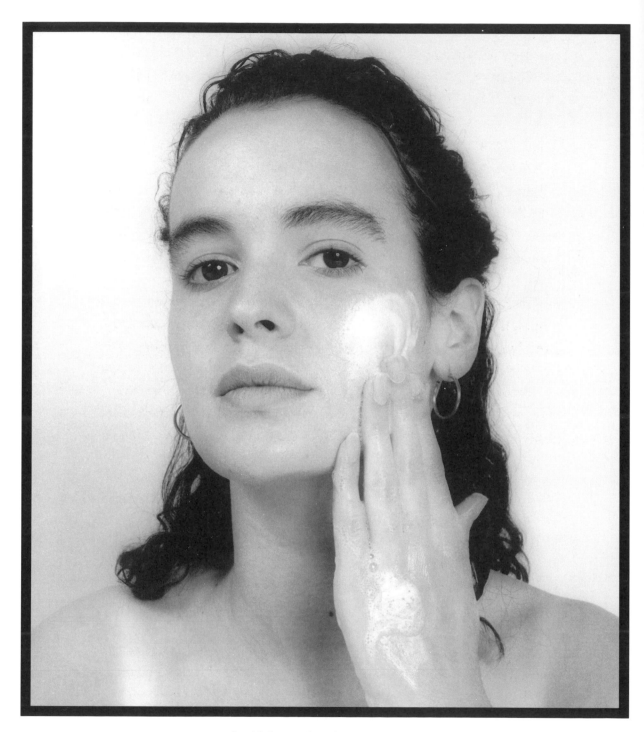

Teenagers should cleanse their skin with a mild facial wash.

lotion can be applied in the morning if desired, but only to the neck and the outside of the face, not to the T-panel.

For boys the daily routine should also be simple. Boys will be beginning to shave and can develop skin irritations if they are too rough with the razor. I think a facial wash is best to use before shaving. This type of product is formulated to prevent too much disturbance of the skin's pH factor (acid balance) and will help keep the skin soft. Many of the products on the market are in bottles suitable for use by boys and girls. After shaving, a little moisturizer on the area will help prevent shaving rashes.

Teenage skin: dry/sensitive

A young skin should not be dry or sensitive. If you are unfortunate enough to have some sensitivity, stop using the products you currently use. Your body is becoming sensitive to its own immune system and is reacting to chemicals in the creams.

Also check that your diet is balanced (see page 15). It is important for young, growing adolescents to eat properly. Many girls are concerned about their weight and they begin to diet badly, without a proper understanding of nutrition. The result is a lack of vitamins which reflects in dry skin and brittle hair and nails. Stress also plays a

> ❛ *A young skin should not be dry or sensitive.* ❜

vital role in how skin reacts to pressure, whether from examinations, emotional upheavals or the strain of a first job. A vitamin and mineral supplement taken at this time will help to restore the balance, but do try to and treat the body as a whole and not in isolated compartments. Remember, if you feel good, you will look good.

To look after a dry and sensitive skin you should use only unperfumed products. Do not use any toners, fresheners or face masks, and avoid sunbathing. Use moisturizer if required, but if the dryness is extreme try a facial massage (see page 49) with evening primrose oil on the dry areas.

Don't feel that you simply have to accept having dry, sensitive skin; it is not a normal condition for young skin. At least at this age it should correct itself with careful handling.

ADULTHOOD (TWENTIES, THIRTIES AND FORTIES)

Usually, by the time you are an adult, your skin will have settled down, and your skin type will be either dry/sensitive, normal/combination or greasy. Male skin will almost certainly have settled down by now because it is thicker and hormonal balances will have adjusted to manhood. The following advice relates to women, but in fact men could follow the same routines.

Adult skin: dry/sensitive

A dry or sensitive skin can be caused by genetic considerations or damage due to neglect. Some types of sensitivity are aggravated by stress and by cosmetics that irritate the skin and cause allergic reactions.

> *Sensitivity is usually caused by the continual use of the wrong products and ignoring the warning signs.*

If you have taken care of your skin from adolescence, by the time you reach your middle years you should only be dealing with 'genetic' dryness. The easiest way to combat this is by avoiding using water or any treatments that might dry the skin out. Weather conditions can have a damaging effect so keep it protected. Make-up is a tremendous help in this respect because a cream or liquid foundation is a moisturized base with colour pigment added. If your skin is very dry, you will need an untinted moisturizer beneath.

Sensitivity is a problem that is usually caused by the continual use of the wrong products and ignoring the warning signs of tingling and irritation until the skin has become sensitive to its own immune system. To overcome this, you must stop using all products and then, one by one, re-introduce them to the skin until it once again establishes its own protective barrier. It is better to leave off the original products and re-introduce them at a later date.

Usually, an allergy to a certain brand does not mean the brand is not good. It is just that your particular skin is 'sensitive' to one of the

> **❝ The more gently dry skin is handled, the better it will respond. ❞**

ingredients in that specific brand. However, when you have a breakdown in the skin's immune system, the product that has caused the irritation may not be the originator of the disorder; it is usually only the trigger. Many people with this kind of condition are highly strung and under stress, for a variety of reasons. They keep their problems inside and are unable to discuss them. This can, like the final straw, cause the skin to over-react.

I have found that the following regime works best for a skin that is dry or sensitive.

Cleanse the skin with a cleansing cream (preferably unperfumed or only very lightly fragranced). Work it well into the face and neck, then remove it with tissues. Repeat twice if you are wearing make-up; in the morning once is sufficient. Wipe over the face with pads of cotton wool soaked only in tepid water or rosewater. Do not use a toner or freshener as these can dry out the outer layer faster than you would wish. Do not use a scrub, washing gel or face mask.

Great care is the key to looking after this type of skin. The more gently it is handled, with rich, emollient creams and gentle massage, the better it will respond. It will reward you with a good colour tone and with softened lines.

Use a conditioning cream regularly, working it well into the skin in circular movements and leaving it to soak in for at least ten minutes before gently blotting away any surplus with a tissue. Do not go to bed with cream on your skin because it will only cause swollen eyes and, over a period of time, make the skin 'heavy'. Skin is a living thing and needs to be able to function. The slight amount of oil the skin takes in is absorbed within ten minutes; anything left on the skin is surplus to requirements.

Sensitive skin types are in need of continual protection and a moisturizer is always necessary. Be careful, however, when buying this type of product: many now contain sun filters, which can be irritants to the person with sensitive skin.

Adult skin: normal/combination

This type of skin is a blessing. The T-panel is neither too oily nor too dry, and the surrounding areas are soft and unlined. The skin feels soft to the touch. Usually this type of skin has been trouble-free and,

> **' I have never seen a neglected skin that did not respond well to regular skin care. '**

although by the forties there are a few lines around the eyes, it still looks good.

If combination skin has been neglected in earlier years, it may have developed open pores or, at worst, congested pores, but this can be remedied by a good skin care routine. I have never seen a neglected skin that did not respond well to regular skin care. But you do need to follow the routine very conscientiously, in order to prevent excessive drying out in later years, especially after the menopause.

Once a month, have a facial, at a good beauty salon, or carry out the routine for a facial given on pages 45–51. Every morning, cleanse with a non-alkali soap or facial wash and water, and every evening use a cleansing milk or cream followed by a mild tonic to remove the traces of cleanser. Follow these guidelines for cleansing and you will see a change of tone and increased clearness.

Moisturize just the outsides of the face and neck, leaving the T-zone free. (Allowing it to function freely will result in this area looking more refined.) Do not forget to moisturize your neck, which because of its lack of oil and sweat glands ages quicker. Use a conditioning cream two or three times a week, massaging in the cream and leaving it for about 10 minutes before blotting away any residue. Do not go to bed with conditioning cream on your skin.

Adult skin: greasy

Greasy skin looks heavy and unrefined, with open pores. The use of moisturizers on the T-panel may have been the cause of the open pores; if this is the case, it should be stopped immediately. Pores cannot be closed from the outside, but they will close by themselves if allowed to do so.

If the skin has been neglected, the pores will have become badly

> **6** *Pores will close by themselves if allowed to do so.* **9**

congested in the T-panel. The first thing to do is to clear this out. It cannot be done with harsh scrubbing methods, however. Instead, clean the skin thoroughly, morning and night, with a good cleansing milk followed by a gentle facial wash.

Greasy skin is not usually prone to wrinkles. Its main problem is the possibility of whiteheads (milia) which occur under the skin. I have known assistants on beauty counters tell customers that these are acid spots, but I can assure you they are not. They are tiny plugs of solidified oil which have to be removed with a sterile needle and a blackhead extractor. They usually occur when there is too much oil in the pore and the outer, horny layer of skin is not shedding off as efficiently as it should.

This skin type will benefit from a weekly face mask (see pages 45 and 50). If possible, have a professional facial once a month, but make sure that the beautician does not squeeze your skin.

During the menopause, greasy skin can develop mature acne. If this should happen to you, see your doctor for a course of antibiotics to help slow down the oil glands. You might even be tested for menopausal symptoms and put on a course of Hormone Replacement Therapy (see page 101), which can improve the skin by preventing pustulation and smoothing it out.

THE YEARS AFTER FIFTY

By the fifties, even an oily skin will be starting to dry out naturally. Mature skin can still have a lively look to it but you should expect to see a few lines and some broken capillaries, which will be more pronounced on fair skin. If you do have any broken capillaries, I suggest you avoid any salon treatments which involve heat, such as diathermy and cathiodermie. They can damage the skin by increasing the blood flow too quickly, putting a strain on weak blood vessels.

Mature skin: normal

Always protect normal skin in cold or windy weather, and stay out of the sun as much as possible. Use a sun protection product (see page 104) but do be careful about applying it to the centre panel, as it could create tiny oil spots. Leave it for a few minutes then blot away any excess. You will still be protected because the cream, together with its screen, will have been slightly absorbed into the skin.

Use a gentle cleansing lotion or cream morning and night. Never use a toner, but a final rinse with lukewarm water is all right if your skin can take it. Nourish the skin daily with a conditioning cream to keep it soft – this is what is sometimes called night cream but should not be used just before you go to bed. Instead, find a time convenient to yourself. After cleansing, massage the conditioning cream well into the face and neck. Allow it to be absorbed, then blot away any excess after ten minutes. Use moisturizer as a daily protection, and keep everything simple and gentle. Do not use face masks or, if you feel you must, not more than once a month.

When people start to take care of their skin gently, instead of scrubbing away at it, I often notice a tremendous improvement — wrinkles soften and lines ease out. The skin begins to radiate a glow.

Mature skin: dry/sensitive

This type of skin occurs post-menopause, as the lack of oestrogen and the gradual breakdown in the skin's natural responses begin to show. Fine lines appear, the skin lacks lustre, and brown spots and skin tags develop. Nevertheless, many of my clients who possess this skin type

❛ When people start to take care of their skin gently, instead of scrubbing away at it, I often notice a tremendous improvement. ❜

still look good. They have managed to take care of themselves to the point that the lines have been kept soft, and the skilful use of make-up helps to conceal irregularities of colour and texture.

Skin in this age group does not have a great amount of oil and sweat to assist in the softening and protecting job, so it is very important to 'feed' the skin with softening and protecting creams. Never use skin fresheners, scrubs or drying face masks. A simple but effective routine is to use a cleansing cream, rather than a lotion, twice in the evening and once in the morning, massaging it well into the face and neck, then removing it with tissues. If you wish, use a little luke-warm water with a facecloth to remove the greasy feel at the end of the cleansing cycle. Massage in a conditioning cream. Creams containing vitamins E and A are particularly beneficial because both vitamins are oil-soluble and therefore penetrate the skin very slightly to make it soft. A moisturizer should be used during the day.

SKIN CARE ROUTINES

		TEENAGE SKIN				ADULT SKIN (20s, 30s, 40s)			MATURE SKIN	
		Dry/Sensitive	Normal	Greasy	Blemished	Dry/Sensitive	Normal/Combination	Greasy	Dry/Sensitive	Normal/Combination
Non-alkali soap/ facial wash	am		X	X	X		X	X		
	pm			X	X			X		
Cleansing lotion	am	X								X
	pm	X	X				X	X (If wearing make-up)		X
Cleansing cream	am					X			X	
	pm					X			X	
Skin freshener	am									X
	pm							X		X
Warm water rinse	am	X				X			X	
	pm	X	X			X	X		X	
Moisturizer	am	X	X			X	X		X	X
	pm									
Conditioning cream	am					X				
	pm						X		X	X
Kaolin face mask (page 50)	am (once a month)			X	X (only if done by a beautician)		X	X		X (optional)

QUESTIONS FROM CLIENTS

Do I need to use eye make-up remover before cleansing?

Eye make-up remover is not necessary, as cleansers will adequately break down the waterproof ingredient in eye make-up. (Contact lens wearers, however, prefer to use non-oily products to prevent the lenses from smearing.) Eye make-up should be removed prior to cleansing the rest of the face. The correct method is to take some cleansing lotion or cream on to the finger and thumb, and 'scissor' mascara off the eyelashes, then wipe it away with cotton wool impregnated with the cleanser. Finally, cotton wool that has been soaked in warm water and pressed out is wiped over the eye area.

My friend's acne cleared up a lot after a holiday in the sun. Would that work for mine too?

I just wonder if your friend has acne? Acne is due to a hormonal imbalance and therefore cannot be cured by the sun. However, the sun is a drying agent and can dry out the top layer of skin, and it is quite true that a small amount can appear beneficial to skin that is blemished. Nevertheless, great care must be taken to avoid burning the skin and thereby exacerbating the condition because the skin can harden and prevent the oil from escaping sufficiently, making it more prone to bacterial invasion. Doctors in the past used to prescribe drying agents for this type of condition until it was realized that too much drying out of the top layer only led to oil glands becoming over-activated, and thereby blocking the pores. My advice would be a little sun, but no more.

How do you apply cleanser and moisturizer?

Wash your hands and then pour a small quantity of cleanser into your hand. With a washing action, apply to cheeks and neck and work up to the forehead in circular movements just as you would if you were washing your face with soap. Work it well in; the warmth of the fingers will help it penetrate slightly. Remove with tissues and repeat the whole process for a second time. Take care to work it into the nose and chin area so that you can unclog any stale oil. Finish with warm water and a cloth and then towel dry. If you are very dry-skinned you can omit the water at the end of the cleansing routine.

Moisturizer should be applied sparingly and not on the centre of the face. This 'T' zone has many millions of oil and sweat glands and does not require additional moisture unless you are elderly or have been ill. If in doubt, leave it out! It should be applied to the neck and, if necessary, to the outer corner of the eyes with the middle and ring fingers of both hands. Do not forget to blot with a tissue if you think you have used too much.

Does moisturizer add water to the skin ?

The simple answer is no. Moisturizer consists of about 80 per cent water and 20 per cent oil. This formulation acts as a waterproof coat to the skin, preventing oil and sweat from evaporating too quickly. That is why it is important not to use moisturizer on the active part of the face – the central area known as the T-zone – which would stop the body from functioning correctly. What many beauty books do not tell you is that the skin is a living, functioning organ and if it requires more moisture it will provide it – especially if you do not neglect it.

THE JANET FILDERMAN

HOME FACIAL

Supplement your daily skin care routine with a monthly home facial. It will cleanse deep down into the pores, soften the skin, temporarily boost the circulation and give your complexion a healthy glow. (It should not be used, however, if you are suffering from acne.) The steam treatment in step 2 is used for only a few seconds, to make your skin more receptive to the facial. However, it is not suitable for anyone with broken capillaries or damaged skin (specifically, anyone suffering from sunburn, pustules, rashes, open sores, cold sores, rosacea or psoriasis).

◆

Items required:
Cleanser
Tissues
Facial sauna or large bowl
Large towel
Blackhead extractor
Magnifying glass
Cotton wool buds
Surgical spirit
Conditioning cream
Cotton wool squares
Kaolin mask, made up as follows: 5 ml/1 teaspoon
Fuller's earth or kaolin powder (available from
chemists), mixed with a little distilled water to the
consistency of single cream
6mm/¼ inch paintbrush
Eye lotion
Timer
Moisturizer

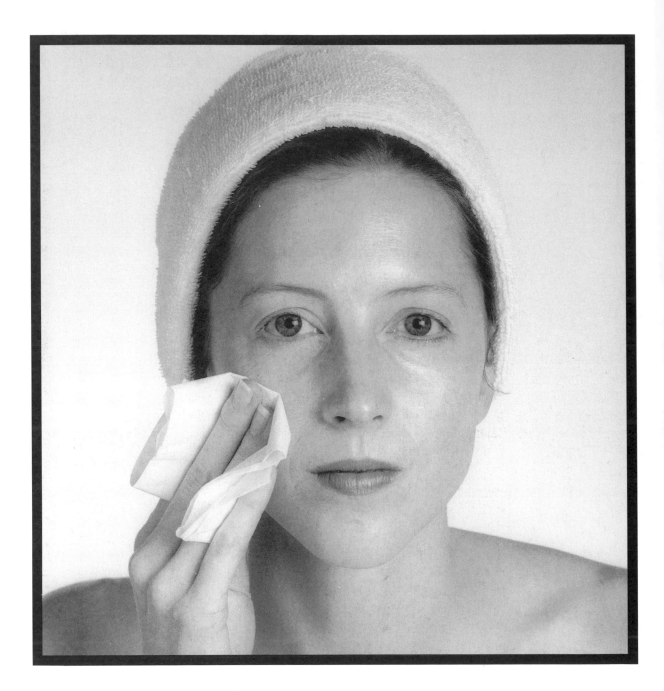

1 Clean face and neck thoroughly with cleanser (as described on page 44). Wipe it off with tissues.

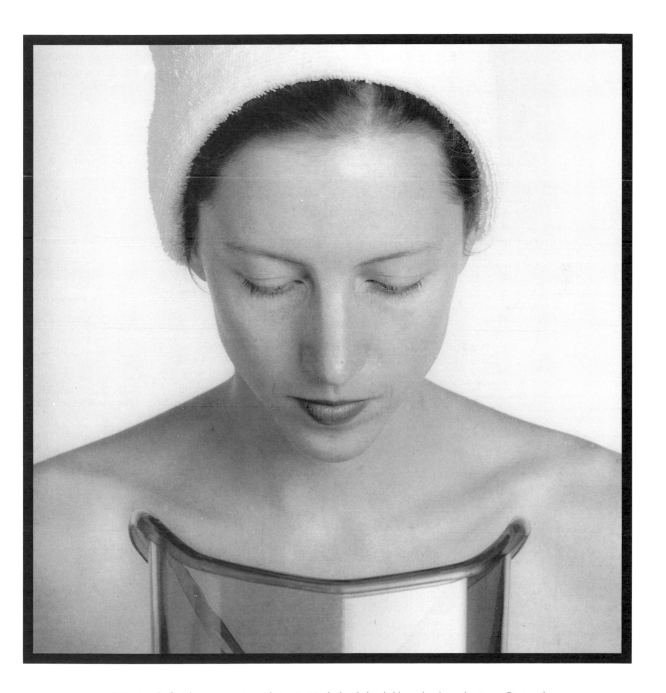

2 Heat up the facial sauna, or put some hot water into the bowl, then hold your head over the steam. Cover with
a towel. You should remain over the steam for only a few seconds, in order to soften the skin.

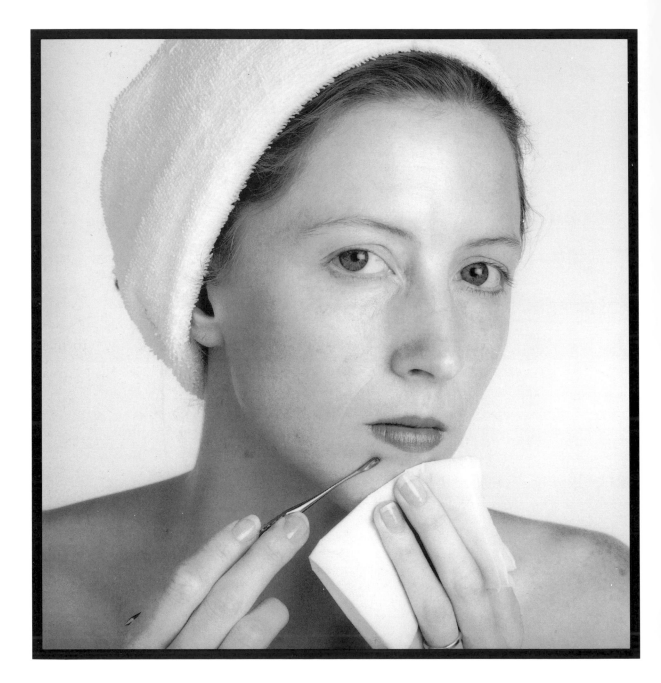

3 Dry your skin with tissues. Holding a tissue in one hand and using a blackhead extractor, position the hole over a congested pore, and press gently. The stale plugs of oil will come out through the hole in the extractor. Do not press over a spot. Work your way round the face, using the magnifying glass to locate small blocked pores. The centre of the T-panel will be the main problem area, but you should also check around the ears. When the process has been completed, treat each spot individually by dabbing it with a cotton wool bud soaked in surgical spirit.

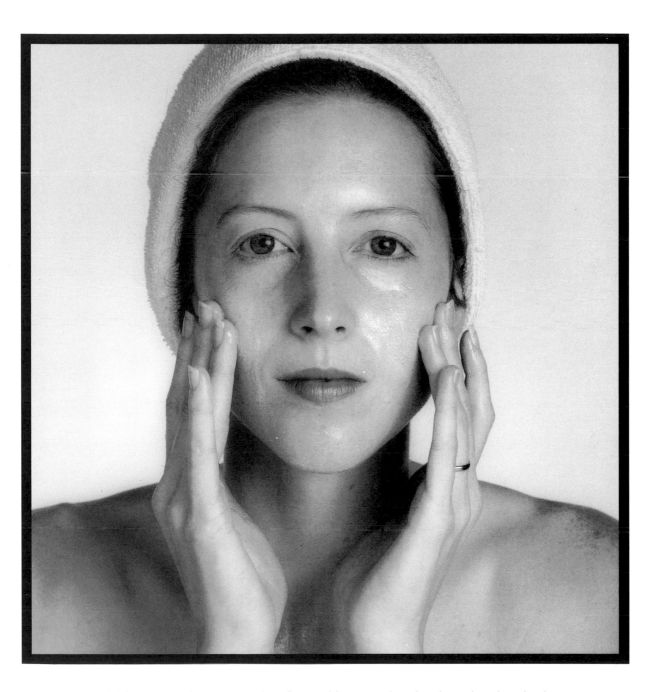

4 Take up some conditioning cream with your fingers and, beginning at the neck, work up and over the neck and face. Use slow, circular movements and work in around the eyes. Finish off across the forehead and then repeat the process, once again working from the neck upwards. Blot with a tissue and, using pads of cotton wool soaked in tepid water, remove any surplus cream from the neck and face.

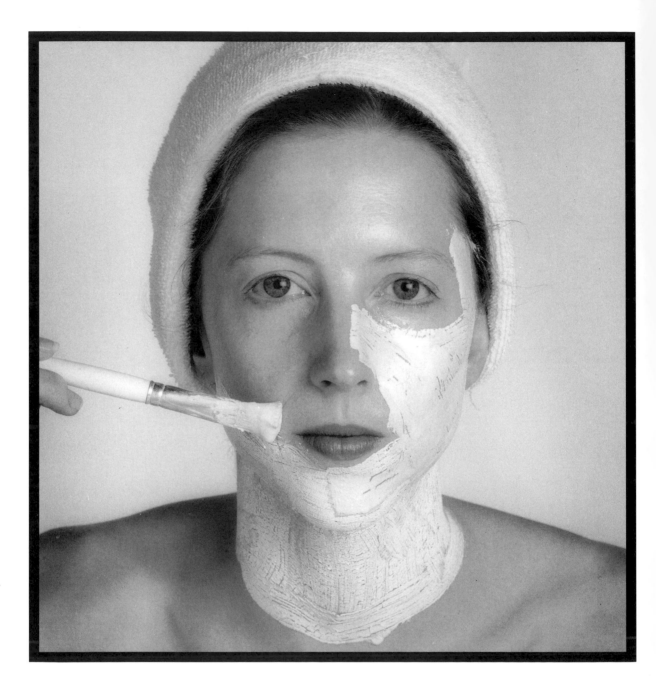

5 Make up the mask as described on page 45 and, with the clean paintbrush, apply it over the face and neck. Kaolin and Fuller's earth have the effect of degreasing and unblocking pores. Place a pad of cotton wool, soaked in eye lotion, over each eye and rest for ten minutes with the mask on your skin. It is best if you take a kitchen timer with you so that you have a chance to relax.

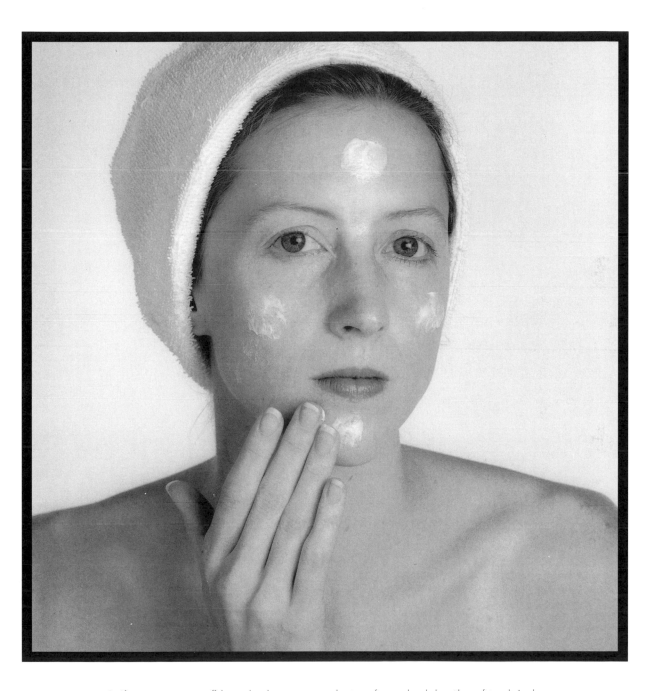

6 After ten minutes, rinse off the mask with warm water and pat your face and neck dry with a soft towel. Apply a little moisturizer to the neck and outer sides of the face.

CHAPTER THREE

BODY GROOMING

Most women concentrate their skin care on the face, but body skin also needs gentle, effective care. In fact, body grooming provides ideal opportunities for pampering oneself – something which every woman should make a regular part of her life.

BATHING

Bathing (or showering) is obviously the focus of body skin care, but let me first of all warn you that it is possible to have too much of a good thing. Over-frequent bathing can dry out the skin, especially in winter, and particularly if the water is too hot. Water ideally should be about body-temperature: just under 38°C/100°F. Water that is too hot dries out the skin badly and may lead to broken capillaries in people who already have weak capillary walls. It can also make you feel tired and faint and can even put a strain on your heart and circulatory system. Long soaks are to be avoided, too, as they temporarily dehydrate the skin, so limit your bathing time to ten to twenty minutes.

The hardness of the bath water is another factor. Soft water is preferable for cleansing, because the interaction of hard water and soap creates a residue on your skin that is difficult to rinse away and can be irritating and drying. Therefore, an additive that softens the

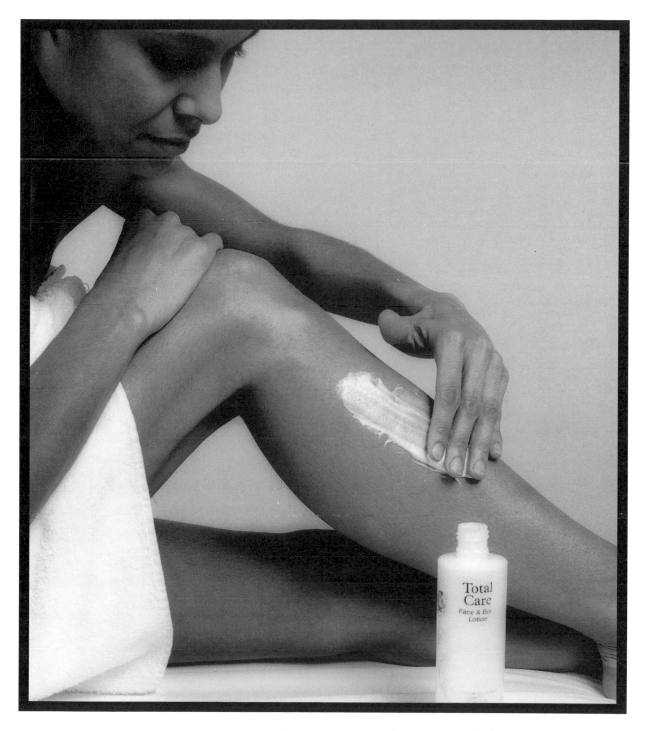

Legs and arms are prone to dryness, so use a good moisturizer regularly.

water is important. Incidentally, if you do use soap, choose a transparent glycerine soap, which is less drying than other types.

Bath/shower additives

There is a wide variety of products available to use in the bath or shower. Probably the best known is foam or bubble bath. This softens and scents the water and does not leave a ring in the tub. Containing a mild detergent, it can be quite drying to the skin, though some contain added moisturizers. Do not use too much, and make sure that it is well mixed with the bath water before you sit down, otherwise it could cause irritation.

Bath and shower gels are similar in formulation to foam baths but are designed to be applied straight to the skin, producing a creamy lather. Shower creams contain extra moisturizers to leave skin soft; they too are applied directly to the skin. Bath milks and creams are added to the bath water to make it soft and creamy, slightly moisturizing the skin without leaving an oily residue.

Bath salts or crystals are basically fragranced and coloured water softeners. They can, however, be drying and so should be avoided if you have dry skin.

Bath oils are added to the bath water not to cleanse but simply to help moisturize the skin. There are two types: those that disperse in the water and those that float on the surface. The dispersing type (which are basically water softeners and therefore make the skin feel softer) are more popular, as they do not leave a ring in the tub. But if you have dry arms and legs, I would suggest you use the type that float on the surface of the water, as they cling to the skin, coating it in an invisible film of oil. (Be careful not to rub it all off with the towel after bathing, however.) You can make your own version of the floating type of bath oil with sunflower oil to which you add a few drops of essential oil in a fragrance of your choice. If you have oily skin or are prone to spots on the back, bath oils are not really suitable, as they could make your skin oilier still.

Bath capsules are dispersing bath oils in gelatin form, which dissolve in hot water. They generally contain a higher proportion of fragrance than liquid bath oils do.

BODY LOTIONS

Arms and legs are usually the first parts of the body to show signs of dryness, often as early as childhood, and the regular use of a good moisturizer or conditioning cream will help to keep the skin soft and smooth. The oils and creams used in the bath/shower help somewhat but are not sufficient in themselves.

Many, many of the skin care creams and lotions that are available are duplicated over and over again, and it is certainly not necessary to

> *Different creams for the cheeks, eye area, neck and body are not necessary. If it is good enough to soften the cheek, it will be good enough to soften skin generally.*

use different creams for the cheeks, eye area, neck and body. If a product is good enough to soften the cheek it will be good enough to soften skin generally. If you have a drawerful of creams, I suggest that you use each one up and then stick with just one good moisturizer or nourishing cream. Use it frequently. I know that getting ready in the morning is already hectic enough, but it really will help to keep your skin soft and in good condition.

ELBOWS, KNEES AND HEELS

Exfoliating creams or scrubs for the body, like those for the face, are used to remove surface cells and create smoother skin. Unfortunately, they can also cause sensitivity when used incorrectly, and I feel that it's best just to use these products to treat the rough skin on elbows, knees and heels. A sponge or flannel is effective enough for the rest of your body.

Areas of thick, rough skin can be a problem. The skin on elbows and knees thickens as a result of time spent leaning or kneeling on them, while ill-fitting shoes or sandals with straps can cause the skin on heels to become rough or hardened and even to crack. All these areas will benefit from the use of a scrub cream, coarse sea salt, a pumice stone or a loofah to slough off some of the thick, dry cells on the surface.

Greyish-looking elbows can be lightened by cupping them in lemon halves for five minutes two or three times a week, as the lemon juice has a slight bleaching effect. Or you could combine exfoliation

> ❛ *Save your scrub creams for elbows, knees and heels. They may cause sensitivity when used elsewhere.* ❜

and bleaching in one treatment by mixing coarse sea salt with lemon juice and rubbing this into elbows and knees; be sure to rinse it all off thoroughly.

Very grubby elbows can be given the same cleansing treatment as hands with ingrained dirt, described on page 81. After any of these treatments, be sure to apply a generous amount of moisture cream.

BASIC HAND CARE

Everyone loves beautiful hands: perfectly shaped and soft, with strong, healthy nails. Yet hands are extremely vulnerable to daily wear-and-tear, as they are the most hard-worked part of the anatomy. It is amazing that we don't have more problems with them.

Dryness is the fundamental problem affecting hands. This can begin from an early age, which is why it is important to encourage schoolchildren to use a non-alkaline soap such as a transparent glycerine bar and then apply hand cream after washing. Once a child has acquired this habit, it is not difficult to maintain and can prevent much dryness and cuticle damage in later years.

Water can damage skin, and the chlorine and fluoride often added to it now make it even more drying. As much as possible, avoid having your hands in water, especially washing-up water that has a liquid detergent in it – at the same time as the detergent is removing grease from dishes, it is stripping valuable oils from your skin. Use a non-alkaline soap when washing hands. A water softener will also help if you live in a hard-water area.

Wear gloves during cold weather and when doing housework and gardening. Once you are in the habit of slipping them on automatically, it isn't such a nuisance as it seems initially.

Gardening can lead to bacterial invasion of the skin, so guard against it by protecting the hands and cuticles with a barrier cream, even if you use gardening gloves. It will make removing ingrained grime much easier.

Everyone who has to have their hands in water to any extent should use hand cream – or the moisturizer already used on the face and body – to put back the oils that the water has taken out of the skin. There are many hand creams on the market that are light and easily absorbed, leaving no stickiness, so if you have not used one for a long time, try again – you will be surprised. It is a good idea to have one in a pump dispenser by the kitchen sink, so that applying it becomes automatic.

As skin gets older, hands begin to show signs of ageing. Poor circulation may leave them rough and red, or the fingertips bluish in tone. Chilblains too can result from poor circulation (though they are actually most common among young women, when they are due to an exaggerated and uncoordinated response by the blood vessels in the skin to a lowering of temperature). Poor circulation may also cause nails to develop ridges or to break through lack of nourishment.

Brown spots often appear on hands, and the knuckles swell. Dryness will be a continual problem, no matter how much cream you massage in. But do persevere for it will certainly make some difference.

NAIL CARE

Well cared-for nails are an intrinsic part of lovely hands. Nails are made of keratin – the horny, protective layer of the skin formed from the skeletons of epidermal cells as they grow, mature and die.

Caring for cuticles

With nails, the major problem is caused by dryness of the cuticle, the crescent-shaped shelf of skin at the base of each nail. It protects the matrix, a spongelike substance beneath the skin consisting of the

> *With nails, the major problem is caused by dryness of the cuticle.*

cells that will ultimately become the new nail. For the new nail to be healthy, care must be taken not to damage these cells. When they begin to grow on to the nail bed, they have to pass through the cuticle; if it is hard, dry or tight on to the nail bed, the new cells become misshapen and ridged. This is the beginning of nail damage.

All nails are tender and easily damaged. It is not until a nail grows beyond the finger that it hardens and dies. Consequently, it is vital that the cuticle is gently creamed and eased back from the nail bed with a hoof stick (a rubber-tipped orange stick) on a daily basis, to allow the young cells to develop.

Use a good cuticle cream each night before going to bed, working it well into the cuticle. Pick up the cream on the end of a cuticle stick so that you can apply it more accurately to the cuticle and will have a free thumb to work the cream into the area. Alternatively, you could try a cuticle pen, which is exceptionally easy to use.

Whenever you apply hand cream, massage some of it into your cuticles. Also, a bath will make cuticles easier to push back, so when you are drying yourself afterwards, gently push them back with the towel.

Cutting the cuticle incorrectly (see page 64) can lead to fungal or bacterial infection. Many nail biters bite the cuticle as well, and I know of people who have developed a nail infection as a result. Even just picking at the cuticle can cause damage such as ridging to the nail.

Enamels, removers and hardeners

Nail enamels and varnish removers will not do you any harm under most circumstances. Remember, however, that the acetone in varnish remover is very drying to nails and cuticles, so choose an oily one or a non-acetone-based remover, and use it sparingly and as infrequently

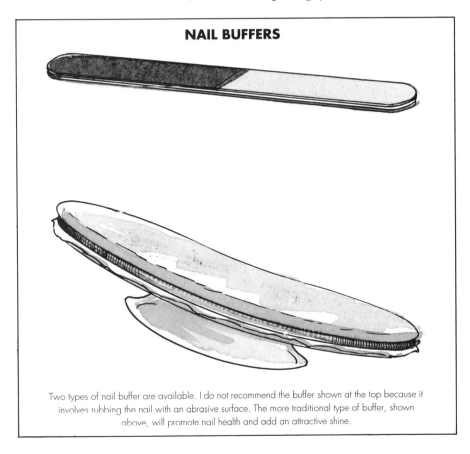

NAIL BUFFERS

Two types of nail buffer are available. I do not recommend the buffer shown at the top because it involves rubbing the nail with an abrasive surface. The more traditional type of buffer, shown above, will promote nail health and add an attractive shine.

as possible. Using a non-chip formulation of nail enamel, which contains silicone, will make a manicure longer-lasting, and also easier to retouch, so that remover does not have to be used so often.

Some nail product ingredients can cause allergies. Formaldehyde resin, for example, which is found in many nail hardeners, can occasionally cause rashes on the fingers or around the eyes (as a result of small particles entering the air after buffing or filing nails or blowing on nail enamel to dry it). If you have noticed any such irritation, it may well be due to an allergy to nail products.

Never leave chipped varnish on your nails: it looks slovenly and is letting down your image. If the enamel peels too easily, omit it entirely, in favour of a good buffing which will bring out the natural shine in your nails. Clean, clear nails are better looking than chipped or chewed ones.

Nourishing the nails

Well-shaped, healthy pink nails are undoubtedly attractive. Buffing them gives a natural shine and improves the blood circulation to the nails, thereby bringing more nourishment to the developing cells.

The traditional type of buffer consists of a pad covered with a soft material such as a chamois leather, attached to a handle. It can be used by itself or with a special cream or powder (or simply talc) for extra shine. A newer type of buffer looks rather like a large, smooth emery board, with two or three surfaces of varying abrasiveness, but you should never rub the surface of the nail with anything abrasive and so I do not recommend these.

There has been a lot said about taking gelatin or calcium to promote healthy nails, but the important thing to remember is that cells are renewed by blood supplying amino acids (found in proteins). Therefore, eating a good balanced diet, consisting of sufficient protein, carbohydrate and fat, will have a marked effect. And because I am convinced that we cannot be certain we are taking in all of the necessary nutrients, I recommend you supplement your diet with a daily multi-vitamin and mineral tablet.

THE JANET FILDERMAN

MANICURE

If time or finance prevents you from having a regular monthly professional manicure, do make an effort to take care of your hands and nails at home on a weekly basis. If you are unable to keep varnish in good order, leave the nails clear and buff them instead, following steps two to seven of the manicure. Take time to do the manicure properly, and you will see the rewards in a relatively short time.

◆

Items required:
Tray (to hold all items required)
Nail varnish remover
Cotton wool
Two small bowls, such as plastic food containers
Facial wash
Nail brush
Hand towel
Cuticle oil
Cotton wool buds
Tissues
Hoof stick
Small nail or cuticle scissors
Fine emery board
Hand cream
Optional
Nail buffer
Base coat
Nail colour
Top coat

1 Using varnish remover and cotton wool, remove old varnish from the nails of both hands.

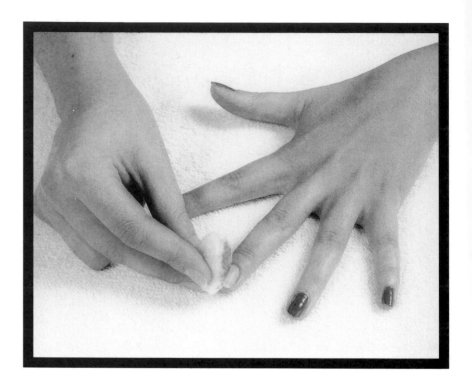

2 In one of the bowls, mix some warm water with a small quantity of facial wash to make a lather. Soak your left hand in this for three minutes, then gently brush the nails with the nail brush. Dry carefully with a soft towel. Repeat for the right hand.

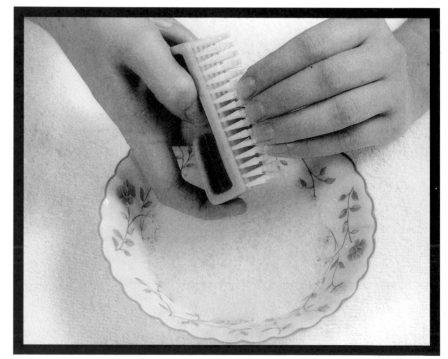

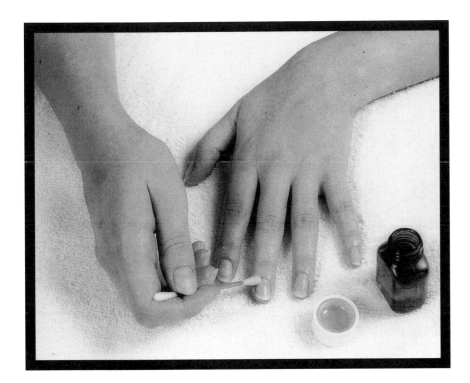

3 Empty a small quantity of cuticle oil into the lid of the bottle and, with a cotton wool bud, apply this to the cuticles of your left hand. Work it well in, first with the cotton wool bud and then with your fingertips. Repeat for the cuticles of your right hand. Discard any cuticle oil remaining in the lid.

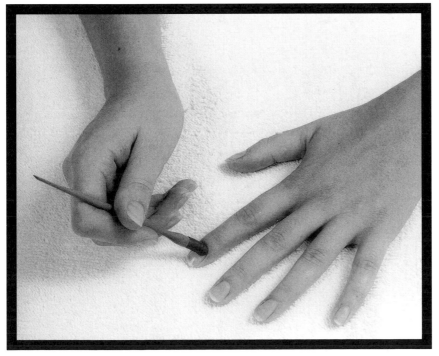

4 Dry cuticles with tissues and then gently push each cuticle back with the hoof stick. Do not worry if it will not go back immediately – it may be too dry, so just do as much as you can.

5 Now use the cuticle scissors to carefully cut away any cuticle that is rough or sticking up from the nail. Leave it alone when the nail and the cuticle look clean and clear. Repeat for the right hand.

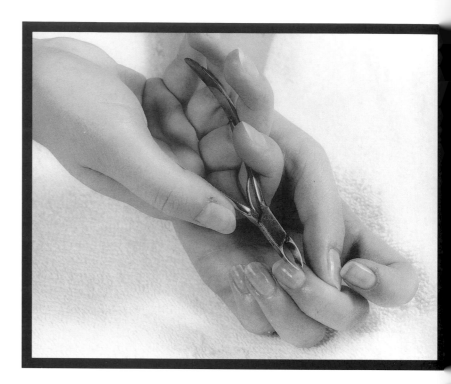

6 Shape the nails of the left hand with the emery board, using only the finer side unless the nails are very hard and out of shape. Work the emery board as if you were playing a fine violin – gently to and fro. Finish off with a downward stroke to take away the fine fibres. The nail shape should be rounded, as it helps to keep the nail strong. Do not take the emery board too far down the nail: give it a side so that the nail is protected. Repeat for the right hand.

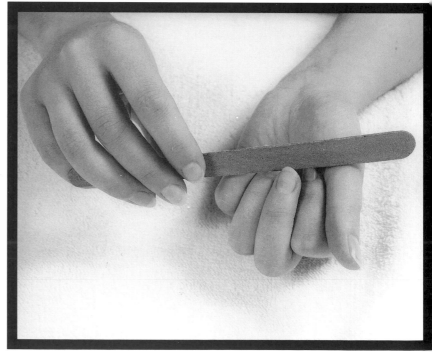

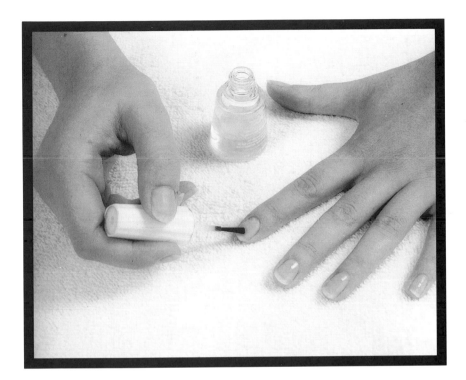

7 Wipe over the nails with cotton wool soaked in nail varnish remover to take off any grease. If you do not normally wear nail varnish, try buffing your nails (see page 60). Otherwise, if you want to paint your nails, now is the time to do it.

First, apply a base coat, which prepares the nail to receive colour, filling out the ridges and allowing the colour to sit well on the nail. Begin with the left hand, wait for a few seconds while it dries and then do the right hand. Wait until the base coat is thoroughly dry before moving on to the next stage.

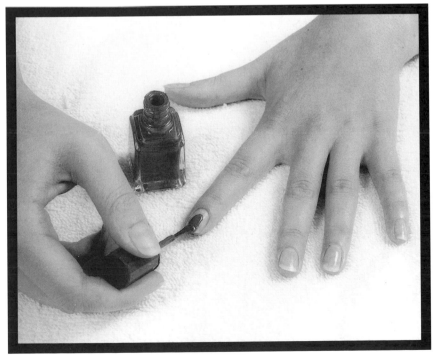

8 To paint your nails professionally, take up some nail varnish on the brush and make a stroke down the middle of the nail.

9 Without taking any more varnish, make a second stroke across the base of the nail. Now take up some more varnish and fill in the two sides of the nail – you may cover some of the centre stroke at the same time. It helps a great deal if you use a table or thick magazine to rest your hand on when you do the painting. Work from index finger to little finger on each hand and only complete the thumbs when the fingers are dry.

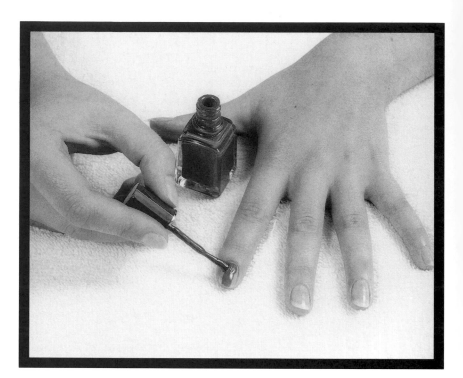

10 The second coat is simply stroked on over the centre of the nail. Impatience is the downfall of the amateur: wait between applications and do not move on to the next stage until the enamel is properly dry. Apply the top coat when the nail varnish is dry. This will give added brilliance of colour and also protect the varnish from chipping.

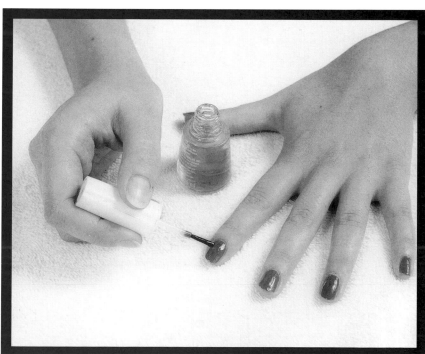

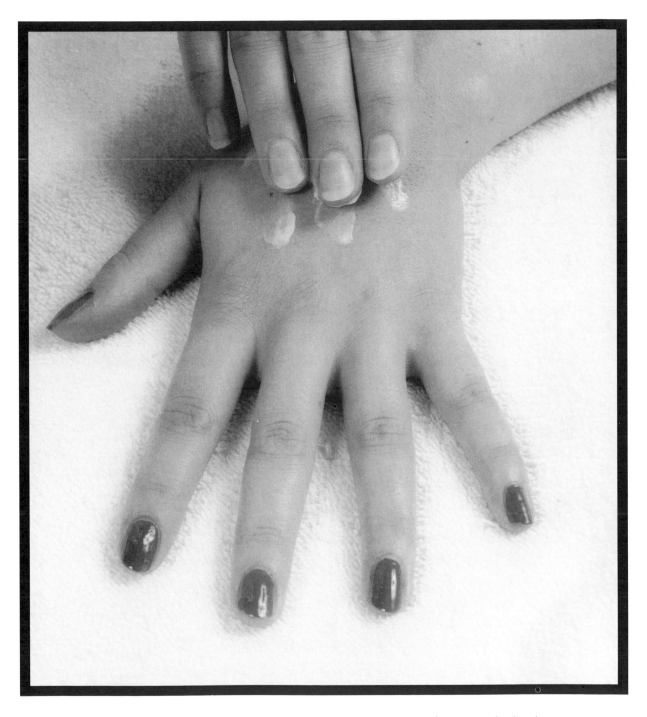

11 When the nails are completed, and perfectly dry, apply a generous amount of cream to your hands and work it well in to finish off your manicure.

CARING FOR YOUR FEET

Feet are the most neglected part of the body. We cramp our toes into ill-fitting shoes, we walk barefoot, we wear sandals that mark our heels and, apart from occasionally cutting our toenails or putting on varnish, we do nothing to care for our feet.

Keeping feet clean, dry and soft is the secret of good foot care. Always dry thoroughly between the toes to prevent fungal infections.

> **❛** *Feet are the most neglected part of the body. Keeping them clean, dry and soft is the secret of good foot care.* **❜**

Regular use of an anti-fungal powder will also help. Scrub cream, a loofah, coarse sea salt or something similarly abrasive can be used to treat rough skin on heels, as advised on page 56. To prevent the problem from recurring, wear shoes that fit properly and will not rub.

When you think of the number of nerve endings in the foot, you can imagine how pain shows in your face when your feet hurt. It affects the way you hold yourself and distorts your spine, throwing it out of line as your body tries to relieve the pressure on the feet. Good feet give good posture.

Two of the most common problems with feet are corns and bunions. Corns are caused because of the pressure of shoes rubbing against the skin. This creates a hardening of the skin, making it dense and thick. You can correct this by gently paring away the hard skin and placing a pad over the area to relieve the pressure, but it will probably return unless you stop wearing the shoes that are causing it. Bunions are caused by the big toe moving too near to the next toe. If this seems to be happening to you, buy a toe separator which will help to keep your big toe straight and prevent damage.

If you have bunions or ingrowing toenails, or badly shaped feet, it is essential to see a qualified chiropodist.

THE JANET FILDERMAN

PEDICURE

It is an unfortunate fact that women may devote hours of care to their make-up, hair and fingernails, then completely forget their feet. Yet a regular pedicure is a must, even if you don't intend to varnish your toenails. Proper foot care will help keep your feet looking and feeling good, improve your posture, prevent snagged tights and bring even greater rewards in old age. So don't wait for summer to start treating your feet to the pedicure described on the following pages.

Items required:

Nail varnish remover

Cotton wool

Washing-up bowl filled with hot, soapy water

Nail brush

Towel

Sharp nail scissors

Cuticle oil

Cotton wool buds

Tissue

Hoof stick

Pumice stone

Base coat

Nail enamel

Top coat

Body lotion

Medicated anti-fungal foot powder

1 Remove old nail polish using nail varnish remover and cotton wool.

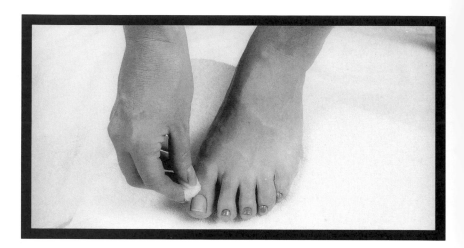

2 Immerse both feet in a bowl of hot, soapy water and soak for five minutes, then scrub toenails with the nail brush. Pat feet dry with a towel, paying particular attention to the area between the toes, where fungal infections can start.

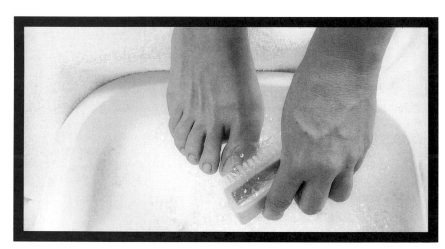

3 With sharp nail scissors, cut the nails straight across. Do not attempt to curve the nail because this can lead to ingrowing toenails.

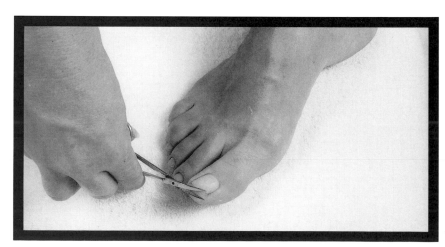

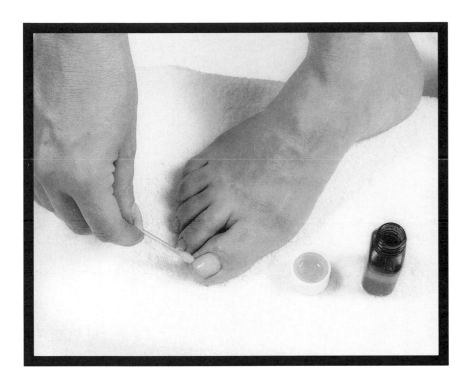

4 Apply cuticle oil to the cuticle of each toe with a cotton wool bud, then work it in with your fingers. The more you do this, the better. Remove any surplus oil with a tissue.

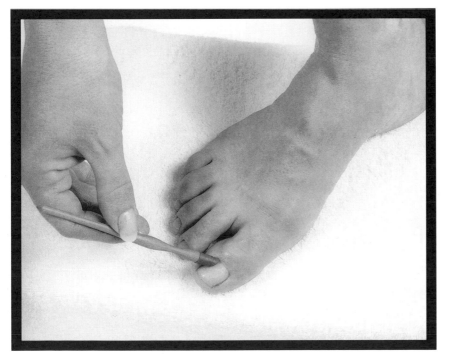

5 Use a hoof stick to gently ease back any cuticle covering the nails. If there is any broken cuticle, remove it with the sharp nail scissors. Work the pointed end of the hoof stick under the nails to remove any debris.

6 If the heels or balls of the feet have any hardened skin, pare this away with the pumice stone.

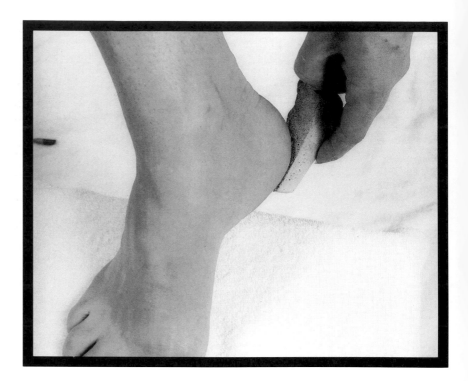

7 Put a pad of cotton wool between each toe and apply base coat to each nail. Allow to dry. Apply nail enamel by painting one thick stroke down the centre and then painting across the nail from left to right. When the enamel is completely dry, apply the top coat to seal and complete the effect. Allow to dry.

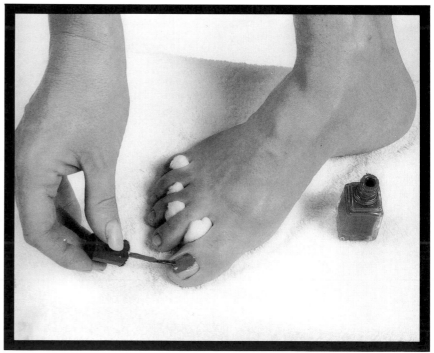

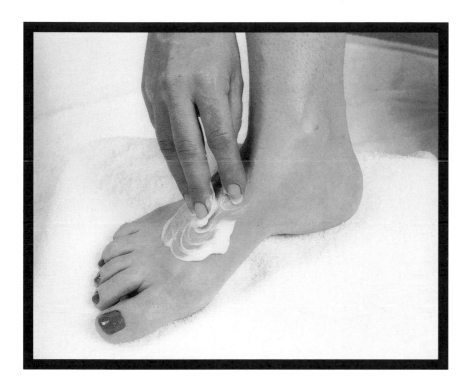

8 When completely dry, apply cream to the entire foot and ankle, paying great attention to the heel – heels need a lot of care if they are to stay soft and free from cracks.

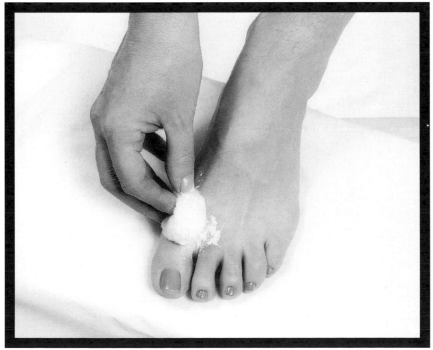

9 To complete your pedicure, put a little anti-fungal powder in the palm of your hand and apply it between the toes with a cotton wool ball, to help combat fungal infection.

HAIR REMOVAL

Although some women have hardly any body hair, or hair that is so fair it is practically invisible, most women have a noticeable amount. Sometimes hormonal changes (during adolescence, pregnancy or the menopause) lead to coarsening of hair or heavier growth where it is not wanted. This might be on the face, nipples or tummy, or excessively on the legs or bikini area. Also, underarm hair is generally removed, which enables deodorants to work effectively.

Excessive hair growth can be embarrassing, ageing and a nuisance.

> **6** *The anguish many women suffer over excessive hair growth is unnecessary, as today there is a variety of methods for removing it.* **9**

I know the anguish women can suffer when they have this problem. Yet, when you consider the range of methods that can be used to remove unwanted hair, this suffering is not necessary – all that is required is a positive approach.

Shaving

Shaving is quick and can be done on the legs and under the arms with little or no problem. Because it removes the hair at skin level, it has to be repeated frequently – in many cases, daily – especially on the legs, and during the summer, when the hair grows faster. Shaving causes the hairs to be prickly to the touch because they are cut off at an angle, leaving sharp ends. It's important to keep the razor in good condition, or hair can become infected with bacteria and the hair follicles can become septic.

Depilatories

Depilatories take a little longer to use than shaving, and some women dislike their strong smell. However, they give a smoother appearance to the skin because the cream travels a little way down the hair follicles and shrivels the hairs just below skin level. As a result, the hairs take slightly longer to appear again. Depilatories can be used on the face as well as the body, but it is advisable to use a cream especially formulated for the face. If you change creams from time to time, you may avoid problems of sensitivity to the chemicals in one particular brand. It is wise to conduct a patch test the day before using a new one. Simply dab a little on the inside of your wrist, then wait 24 hours. If reddening or swelling occurs, do not use it.

Waxing

Waxing can be done at home but it is better done in a salon where the wax can be applied by a professional beautician. Waxing is not quite as simple as it seems. The hair should always be removed in the direction in which it grows, otherwise damage can occur resulting in ingrowing hairs and septic follicles. To tackle the back of your own legs requires you to be something of a contortionist!

If you decide to undertake waxing at home, remember to swab the area with surgical spirit before and after removal of the hair because

> ❛ *Waxing is not as simple as it seems and is best done in a salon. For example, to tackle the backs of your own legs requires you to be something of a contortionist!* ❜

the hair is removed with the bulb which leaves the skin open to bacterial invasion.

There are two types of wax currently available. Hot wax is made from beeswax and is applied directly on to the skin. When it is cool it is pulled off, taking the hair with it. This is now usually only used under the arms and on the bikini line, where the hair is coarser.

More frequently, a cool wax is used. This is made with honey and is warm, sticky and runny. It is applied with a spatula, then a waxed strip of muslin is used to remove the wax and hair.

Bad removal can lead to the hair being broken off at skin level. Regrowth will then be rapid (the same as if you had shaved).

Electrolysis

This is a method of permanent removal of hair and is particularly recommended for hair around the nipples, on the tummy, on the chin or on the upper lip. It involves applying a heat current to the root of the hair with a very fine needle. The root is cauterized, which weakens or kills it; often, more than one treatment is necessary to kill it completely.

Advances in technology have produced faster and more painless

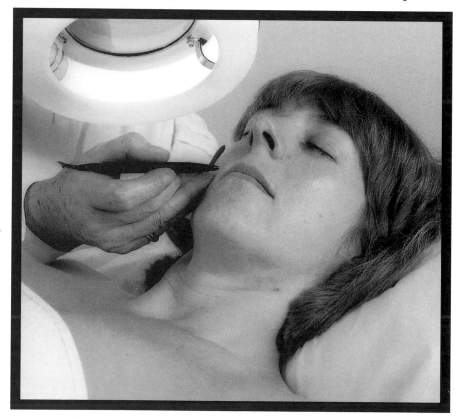

Electrolysis is a method of removing unwanted hair permanently.

methods of permanent hair removal, but it is essential that you visit only a properly qualified electrologist who is a member of the Institute of Electrologists. Scarring and burns can occur in the hands of a poorly trained operator.

Sometimes pimples appear after an electrolysis session, but they will heal within a very short time. The pimples are caused by the body's defence mechanism coming into play. The white blood cells are told to produce pus, which is the body's way of preventing further invasion into an area which – from the body's point of view – is being attacked. When it receives signals that there is no longer a threat, it stops the manufacture of pus, and the pimples disappear.

SAUNAS AND STEAM BATHS

Many people find a sauna or steam bath a relaxing and refreshing way of drawing toxic waste from the body, which is achieved through heavy sweating.

The dry heat of the sauna – usually around 110°C/230°F – is designed to drive out as much of the body's moisture as possible through the skin. In a Finnish sauna, hot stones can if desired be doused with water to create steam temporarily. After about five or ten minutes in the sauna, you go into a plunge pool or cold shower, the effect of which is to stimulate the circulation. Then, if you wish, you repeat the cycle.

Staying in a sauna for too long can cause excessive fatigue or even fainting. At a health hydro I once saw some women who were on a fasting regime being given saunas, and their low blood sugar level was causing them to faint. So be careful, avoid staying in for more than five or ten minutes, and if you have fine skin or broken capillaries, if you suffer from high blood pressure or heart disease, or if you are pregnant or take any sort of medication, don't risk it.

Steam baths are slightly gentler than saunas, as the humidity prevents the heat from drying out the skin in the same way. However, you feel even hotter, because the sweat cannot evaporate from the skin. A session usually lasts for about 15 minutes and is followed by a plunge in cold water.

As with saunas, you should avoid staying in a steam bath for too long and should not use one if you have any of the contra-indications which are listed on the previous page.

AROMATHERAPY

Aromatherapy is a form of facial and body massage using essential oils extracted from plants. Although it has its roots in ancient Egypt and the East, aromatherapy itself was developed in the 1940s and 1950s, after modern distillation techniques enabled chemists to extract the plant essences in sufficient volume.

While its advocates claim that aromatherapy can stimulate the circulation, rejuvenate skin and muscle tissue, reduce inflammation, and improve a variety of conditions (including dry skin and fine wrinkling, greasy skin and acne, cellulite, stretch marks, depression and stress-related conditions such as insomnia, migraine and back pain), I must say that I am sceptical about many of these claims. Nevertheless, in the hands of a skilled therapist it can be a very enjoyable and beneficial treatment.

Aromatherapy is a complex art, and the aromatherapist must be highly trained and experienced not only in using the appropriate massage techniques but also in diagnosing individual needs and mixing exactly the right blend of oils. Incorrect mixing can actually lead to burning of the skin.

The essential oils used are carefully chosen from a range of about 300, each with differing therapeutic properties. The essences are very concentrated and volatile, having been distilled from oils found in the roots, flowers, fruit, leaves, bark or resin of certain plants, such as lavender, sage, geranium, bergamot, sandalwood, basil, eucalyptus, myrrh and ylang ylang. Only pure, naturally occurring oils are used

– synthetic oils have no benefit and can even be harmful. A good therapist blends particular oils to suit your own specific needs, which they must diagnose beforehand. In general, the oils can be grouped into four broad categories: stimulating/reviving, tranquillizing, anti-depressant and anti-inflammatory.

Massage is a fundamental part of the therapy, as it warms the skin, making it more receptive to the oils. Exactly how the oils work in the body is not known, but aromatherapists claim that they work through (a) inhalation, which stimulates the brain and sets off a chain reaction producing physiological effects in the body and (b) rapid absorption through the skin and into the bloodstream.

From my own discussions with doctors and dermatologists, I have concluded that the powerful effects of aromatherapy oils are not due to their penetration of the skin, since skin is a protective organ – one

> **6** *I believe that the benefits of aromatherapy are due to the inhalation of the oils and the massage itself, not to the oils going through the skin into the bloodstream, which I am sure is impossible.* **9**

of its functions is to prevent substances from penetrating it, and it does this extremely effectively. Inhalation, however, is a very plausible explanation. Smell is the most primitive and evocative of all the senses, instantly triggering off strong emotions and physical responses. Massage obviously contributes to the effect too – not only through its deeply relaxing, sybaritic quality but also possibly because of its ability to trigger off the production by the body of endorphins, morphine-like substances which act as natural painkillers and also induce a feeling of wellbeing.

Whatever the mechanism by which it works, an aromatherapy massage by a skilled operator is undoubtedly a delightful experience.

QUESTIONS FROM CLIENTS

I've been thinking about having some false nails. Would they actually protect my own nails?

I am often asked what I think of false nails (either the press-on or the moulded, or 'sculptured' type), and I can only repeat to you what I say to my clients. Beautiful as they are, I would not promote false nails because I have seen some nail beds totally damaged by them. In addition, the nails cannot 'breathe' and become soft and spongey. Some nail additions actually require the real nails to be roughened before the mixture is applied, and this can cause permanent damage.

The types of nail extensions that adhere only to the ends of the nails are not as dangerous as the moulded type. The only problem with these is that you need to learn to use your fingers in such a way as to avoid breaking the extensions, since replacements will be costly.

Should I use a nail hardener?

Nail hardeners come in two types – formaldehyde and resin. Formaldehyde is a chemical which is used to pickle and preserve specimens in laboratories and causes hardening. It can be damaging to surrounding tissue such as the cuticles and, as the nail is still living tissue until it reaches the tip, I would not recommend this type of product.

The other type of hardener, the resins, are like strengthened varnishes and could be used if you have trouble growing your nails to a reasonable length because you often knock them against hard surfaces, for example when typing or playing the piano.

*My nails are rather yellowish looking. What causes this and is
there anything I can do about it?*

Nail enamel can occasionally stain the young nail, turning
it a browny-yellow colour. This condition will only improve
if nail enamel is left off and the new nail allowed to develop
without it.

*How can I make my nails harder and smoother? I've been
told that eating gelatin may help. Or is that just an old
wives' tale?*

I do not think that gelatin will help. Although it contains
protein, it lacks essential amino acids involved in the
formation of keratin, and it has no other nutrients. Keeping
the cuticle free of the nail and healthy is probably the best
course of action. If the nail can grow without having to push
its way past the cuticle, it stands a better chance of being
healthy, and ridging - which is what is stopping your nails
from looking smooth - will not occur. Ridging is often seen
in the nails of older people in particular because their skin
dries out more quickly, and they often neglect their hands
and their diet.

*I do a lot of gardening and can never seem to get my hands really
clean. Do you have any tips?*

If your hands are very neglected, with grime in the grooves,
apply a small amount of industrial cleaner (available from
hardware shops and DIY stores), working it well in. Leave
for ten minutes, then rinse off with warm, soapy water,
towel dry and apply hand cream. (This treatment is also
very effective for elbows.)

I am in my late fifties, and my hands are starting to develop a few brown spots which look rather like large freckles. What can I do to get rid of them?

Brown spots often appear on hands with age. They, can be burned away with dry ice, but this should only be done by trained medical personnel. A bleaching cream (which is also known as fade cream) would have to be used for some time before it would have a noticeable effect on the marks. The active ingredient, hydroquinone, is a strong chemical that is a known skin irritant, often causing redness and irritation, and it also makes the skin photo-sensitive (see page 111). Sometimes the treated skin becomes lighter than the surrounding skin, and the results may be patchy and uneven. Over-the-counter bleaching creams contain a smaller proportion of hydroquinone than do prescription-only bleaching creams, but I feel you should only embark upon this treatment under a doctor's supervision. (For more about bleaching cream, see pages 92–3.) Wearing a sunscreen with a high sun protection factor (see page 104) will help to prevent the formation of further brown spots.

Why do magazines so often recommend applying body lotion to damp rather than dry skin?

The real reason you often see this advice is that the formulation of the body lotion is not efficient enough. As mentioned on page 44, moisturizers are combinations of oil and water, and if the oil is not heavy enough to allow the water to hold on to the skin, the moisturizer evaporates too soon. A lotion containing a lighter-weight oil therefore needs the extra dampness to be effective. Ideally, use a body lotion which does not necessitate this – it will be more beneficial to your skin.

How do epilators work?

An epilator is rather like an electric razor, but it plucks hair out by the roots. It can be painful, but the hairs take longer to grow out than after shaving or using a depilatory, and their regrowth is not prickly. However, it is difficult when using one to avoid breaking the hairs off at the surface.

Would bleaching make the hair on my upper lip less noticeable?

Bleaching is often used on facial hair and forearms, but it is very drying to the skin and tends to make dark hairs look reddish so I do not recommend its use. Instead, you could consider electrolysis, waxing or a depilatory.

What can I do about my varicose veins?

Varicose veins – those knotted, distended, bluish veins that can develop in the legs – are caused by the valves in the veins that lie close to the surface ceasing to work correctly, so that the blood in the veins backs up at these valves. The condition can be hereditary, but pregnancy, the menopause, obesity, bad diet and lack of fibre, standing or sitting still for long periods, lack of exercise, or restriction caused by tight shoes, jeans or pants can make it worse or even trigger it off. See your doctor about them. Depending on the severity of the condition, he may recommend you to a surgeon specializing in the removal of varicose veins. Other measures you can take are to get more exercise; eat more fibre; wear support tights, especially if you are pregnant; and avoid hot baths and restrictive trousers, pants and footwear. Incidentally, the spidery-looking broken capillaries that sometimes appear on the legs are not an early sign of varicose veins.

CHAPTER FOUR

SKIN COUNSEL

Everyone is troubled at some time by skin problems of one sort or another, whether it is the occasional spot or a more permanent disorder. The vast majority of these can be cured, improved or at least disguised effectively.

DRYNESS

If you are young, your skin should not be dry: it is as simple as that. If you do have a dry skin, check whether you are doing something to cause this, and stop using anything that could be the culprit, such as toners, masks or scrubs. Use only cleansers that are unperfumed.

Mature skin needs cleansing cream but not toner. Apply a conditioning cream day and night (blotting off the excess after ten minutes before going to bed). Never leave the skin unprotected: harsh

> *If you are young, your skin should not be dry: it is as simple as that. If it is, check what you are doing to cause this.*

weather and central heating can so easily dry it out. Use make-up or moisturizer for protection during the day.

Check your diet. Perhaps a vitamin deficiency could be the problem. Are you anorexic? Are you a nervous type? All these problems call for medical assistance, so contact your doctor.

OPEN PORES

Open pores do refine with patience and care. They cannot, however, be closed by using astringents. It is the tiny erectile muscles in the skin that control the pores, as part of the body's system for regulating its temperature. If the pores are blocked, the muscles will respond

> *Throw out your astringent – it will make open pores worse.*

by opening the pores wider. Therefore, you must throw out your astringent.

You should also avoid moisturizing this particular area. If your pores are open but clean, the blockage will almost certainly be due to over-moisturizing. If, however, the pores are blocked, then you must get this condition cleared first, using the home facial procedure described on pages 45-51.

SPOTS

Spots are caused by bacteria invading the skin and causing an infection. If you have oily skin and a lot of facial hair, you will probably get spots more often. Acne pustulations and spots are both caused in the same way, but because the oil is waxier with acne, the problem is exacerbated. (Turn to pages 28-31 for specific advice about caring for skin with acne.)

Cleansing skin properly is the key to preventing spots, so follow the skin care advice on pages 28–51 for dealing with your particular skin type. Remember that grease acts like a magnet for bacteria.

To dry out the spot and at the same time kill the invading bacteria, apply a little surgical spirit or liquid antiseptic to the spot, morning and night, until it has cleared. Use a cotton wool bud to apply it, but do not put the cotton wool bud into the bottle of spirit,

> 6 *Never, never squeeze spots, as this will only cause worse problems.* 9

or you could spread bacteria. Instead, pour a small amount into the cap of the bottle, and dip the cotton wool bud in that. Use a new amount of spirit for each application. When you have finished, wash out the cap and replace it on the bottle.

Never, never squeeze spots, as this will only cause worse problems. Squeezing a spot can push a pigment cell into the dermis so that new cells always come out darker when they appear on the surface of the skin. And if there is any facial hair involved, squeezing the spot can result in follicle infection.

BLACKHEADS AND WHITEHEADS

Blackheads and whiteheads can be treated at home if you have a blackhead extractor, but you must be scrupulous about swabbing the area with surgical spirit and also about sterilizing your equipment so that you do not spread germs.

Blackheads are little stale plugs of oil that have failed to reach the surface of the skin. Consequently they stick in the pore and on reaching the air they oxidize and turn black. They can be removed using a blackhead extractor, as explained on page 48. Whiteheads are basically the same thing, but unfortunately they have a keratinized layer of cells between them and the air and therefore stay white. These are the hardest to deal with, and very great care is needed. Swab the area first, then use a magnifying glass to insert a sterilized needle just under the outer layer of cells; this should not draw blood. Next, prize out the milia, which is usually a hard little ball. Finally, swab the area once more.

The regular use of a kaolin mask (see pages 45 and 50) will also

> **6** *Regular use of a kaolin mask will help prevent blackheads and whiteheads.* **9**

help this condition because the chalk in the mask absorbs the stale oil; in light cases it completely cleans out the pore.

Salon treatment consists of vaporization, followed by vacuum suction or extraction, or a combination of both. But do not let a beautician squeeze your skin – it is asking for trouble. Squeezing pushes the problem further into the skin, as explained on pages 32 and 86.

BROKEN CAPILLARIES

Capillaries are the tiny blood vessels that feed the tissues. In later life or if the skin is very fine, the walls of the capillaries may become weakened, then when they dilate excessively they sometimes burst. What you actually see is the blood that has leaked into the surface tissues, not the broken capillaries themselves. Recognizable as tiny red streaks, they occur most often on the cheeks and nose, under the eyes and on the legs. A number of factors can cause the capillaries to dilate excessively – including over-exposure to harsh weather or the sun; drinking alcohol, hot coffee or tea; eating spicy foods; and high blood pressure – but the underlying cause is the weakened capillary walls.

Treatment depends on how bad the capillary damage is. Diathermy, which is a heat current, can be used to cauterize the capillary so that the escaped blood in the surface tissues dries up. The problem is that if the walls of the capillary are already weak, it will probably burst again, possibly in a different place.

There are many cosmetic clinics now set up to deal with this type of condition, but I would recommend that you consult a medically qualified dermatologist first. If you do not wish to bother your own doctor for a referral, a good beautician will be closely involved with one because of her work. At your consultation, find out what the chances are of the problem recurring, and weigh this up against the alternative of concealment with make-up. Sometimes it is better to make the best of a bad job than to encourage further capillary breakdown.

A leading dermatologist advised me that the only real cure for broken capillaries was to strengthen the capillary walls, and he recommended that Rutin, a derivative of vitamin B, be taken every day if a person is known to have weak capillaries. I have seen very good results from this treatment.

ROSACEA

This condition is characterized by acute flushing or redness of the face, which is frequent or even continuous. This is often accompanied by broken capillaries, swelling and sometimes tiny bumps and pustules. It is unusual for rosacea to develop before middle age. Avoiding factors that dilate the weakened capillaries further (such as rapid temperature changes, spicy food, hot drinks and alcohol) will help to control rosacea, but there is no real cure, nor is the actual cause known. Calamine lotion or a mild cream will help to soothe the skin, and in severe cases doctors may prescribe antibiotics to suppress the inflammation. A good make-up base can be used to help camouflage the redness (see pages 124–6).

BLOTCHY SKIN

Blotchy skin is normally due to using the wrong product for a length of time: stop using the products and the condition improves.

Occasionally, however, some skins develop dry itchy patches which are the result of dry eczema. The problem usually flares up when the person is under stress. Anti-histamine creams and tablets will help, and evening primrose oil – taken internally and applied topically – has had good results.

When a skin is sensitive to creams, the last thing you should do is substitute aromatherapy oils or plant extracts. It is not that they are harmful in themselves, but that they are often over-used, which sets up more and more irritation. Concentrated oils can burn, and the mix is very important. I know of an aromatherapist who mixed her own oils and developed burns between her fingers and inside her elbow. Imagine the effect if a lay person mixed her own oils.

E C Z E M A

Eczema can occur at any age and on almost any part of the body. It can be triggered by a nervous disposition or stress. It is a non-contagious allergic and irritant skin condition characterized by dry, scaly, red patches that are extremely itchy. If you suffer from eczema, you have probably found out a great deal more about potential irritants than I could cover in this book. You will probably also know that though eczema cannot be cured, it can be treated. And that means keeping your skin well moisturized and avoiding anything that could irritate it.

Soap and water will irritate your skin, so use a cream cleanser instead, as well as a bland, soothing, conditioning cream. Many ingredients of cosmetic products can irritate the skin or cause an allergy, including fragrance, colouring agents, pearlizing agents, preservatives, lanolin and alcohol. Therefore, it's wise to choose hypo-allergenic products. These do not guarantee that they will not irritate your skin or cause a reaction – they simply reduce the risk. They contain a minimum of known potential allergens and irritants and so are less likely to cause a reaction.

Even water on its own will dry out your skin too much, so use an unperfumed oil or emulsifying ointment in cool water when you bathe. A doctor may suggest you use a low-strength hydrocortisone cream or ointment on the affected parts of your skin or take anti-histamine tablets to suppress the symptoms.

PSORIASIS

Less common than eczema, psoriasis is characterized by irregularly shaped, slightly raised red patches of skin, covered in silvery scales. There is no itching. Common sites are the elbows, knees and the scalp, but it less often affects the face. Psoriasis occurs when the rate of reproduction of the skin cells increases dramatically, and the normally invisible process of discarding flakes of skin becomes noticeable. It is not contagious. Treatment for psoriasis is similar to that for eczema (see page 89). In addition, sunshine is generally beneficial, and preparations containing tar or dithranol are often successful. A doctor may suggest nutritional supplements, ultraviolet therapy or, for more severe cases, certain powerful drugs.

COLLAGEN DAMAGE

This type of deterioration is usually seen on older people but if you have been sunbathing too much it can appear earlier in life. Collagen damage can be recognized by tiny, fine lines running criss-cross on the cheeks and fine lines around the mouth. These should not be confused with lack of muscle tone – for example, lines from nose to mouth and those running across the forehead.

Collagen damage can be corrected on a temporary basis with injections of Zyderm. Zyderm is collagen from cattle (which is very similar to human collagen) mixed with distilled water and is injected within the layers of the skin by a cosmetic surgeon. A scratch test is usually done before treatment to determine whether you are allergic. Immediately after the treatment there is some swelling, but this disappears after a few hours, leaving the facial lines plumped out. The effect lasts for around six months, sometimes longer, then the collagen has to be topped up with further injections. I personally think that using this method too much can eventually stretch the skin.

Using collagen creams can help to keep the skin soft, but it is impossible for the collagen in the cream to be absorbed by the skin.

Some cosmetic surgeons in the United States are using silicone implants to plump out the lines, and I have seen some good results from this. The treatment is not carried out in the United Kingdom.

The acne drug tretinoin, marketed as Retin-A, is now sometimes

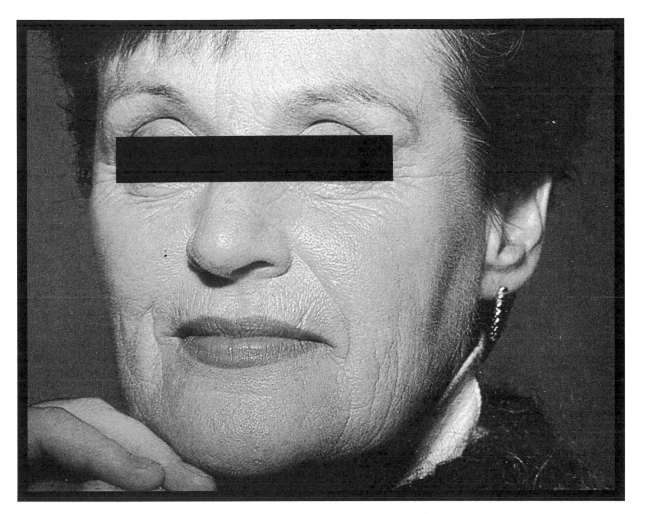

Fine lines around the mouth and on the cheeks indicate collagen damage.

prescribed to reduce facial lines and cross-hatching caused mainly by sun damage, and after several months of treatment the improvement is marked. Its initial side effects are severe, as it causes irritation, inflammation, redness and scaling, but these symptoms disappear after two to ten weeks.

A more serious problem is the fact that Retin-A makes the skin much more vulnerable to the harmful effects of the sun because it lets more of the ultraviolet rays penetrate the skin. Hyper-pigmentation

> ' *The "anti-wrinkle" drug Retin-A makes the skin much more vulnerable to the harmful effects of the sun.* '

(see below) and photosensitivity (see page 111) can result unless a sunscreen with a very high SPF is worn. Also, although acne patients have been using the drug since 1971, the longterm effects of using it to treat wrinkles are not yet known. Not available over-the-counter at present, Retin-A should only be used under a doctor's supervision.

HYPER-PIGMENTATION

This has become more common since the introduction of the birth-control Pill. Hormones and sunlight combine to produce a disturbance of the melanin level and when this occurs, blocks of dark pigment develop in the skin. They usually appear around the eye or mouth but can be anywhere on the body. Changing the type of contraception can improve the condition, but it is important to keep out of strong sun or at least wear a total sunblock.

If you have hyper-pigmentation, consult your doctor. He might suggest that you use a good bleaching cream which is specially formulated to even out the dark patches. A bleaching cream does not significantly fade or bleach skin; it interferes with the production of new pigment, preventing it from surfacing in the treated area. In

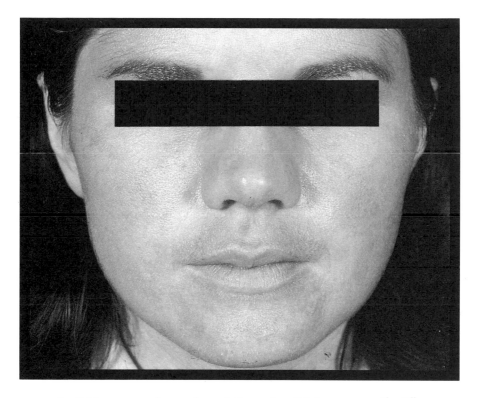

Sunlight may cause hyper-pigmentation such as this in women on the Pill.

time, the darker cells slough off. The active ingredient in bleaching creams is hydroquinone. An over-the-counter cream contains a small percentage of hydroquinone, while a cream prescribed by a doctor or dermatologist may contain a higher proportion.

The first time you use a bleaching cream, do a patch test the day before by dabbing a bit in the crook of your arm. Use the bleaching cream only if there is no redness or irritation within 24 hours.

MOLES

Moles are pigmented growths on the skin. They may be large or small, flat or raised, light or dark. Sometimes hairs grow in them. If you are unhappy with the appearance of a particular mole, or if your clothing is rubbing a mole, it can be quickly and painlessly removed

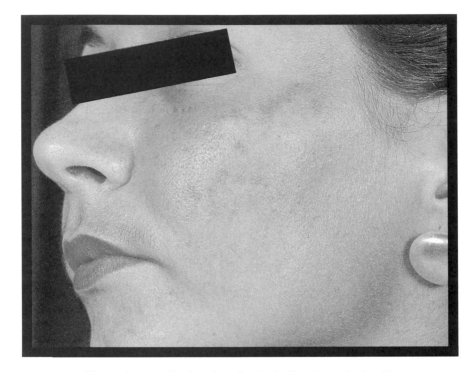

Hyper-pigmentation is a sign of melanin disturbance in the skin.

by a doctor or dermatologist. Once removed, moles generally do not grow back.

Moles are usually harmless. But with the growing incidence of skin cancer, it is wise to check them regularly. If a mole changes in size or colour, becomes itchy or begins to bleed, see your doctor straight-away. Early treatment of cancerous moles – known as malignant melanomas – is essential.

SKIN TAGS

These are tiny, wart-like tags that usually appear on the neck and under the arms when one is getting older. They can be removed by an electrologist or dermatologist. You could also use a product that is available for wart removal. In order to use this correctly, you should paint the surrounding skin with petroleum jelly before applying the product. Repeat the treatment daily until the skin tag has burned away.

Two old 'home' remedies are to rub lemon juice over the area, or to wet the sulphur end of a match and rub that on the affected area. These treatments are done twice a day until the tag drops off. I believe they work for some people – they will do you no harm if they do not work for you.

DARK UNDER-EYE CIRCLES

Dark circles under the eyes usually accompany olive skin. They become more intense when a person is unwell and are usually accompanied by dark eyelids. I do not know of any treatment available for this condition but it can be minimized by concealing cream and skilful use of make-up (see page 124–6).

Some dark circles on light-coloured complexions are the result of lack of sleep or illness; these tend to look bluer in tone. The treatment is the same. However, in this case the condition usually improves as the health gets better, for the problem is not one of pigmentation but of stress.

PUFFY EYES

Puffy eyes are generally caused by leaving creams on the face overnight, which tends to block the lymph nodes by the eyes and thus prevent them from discharging fluids. Even cleansing lotion that is not removed properly can lead to puffy eyes. Therefore, after your night-time cleanse with cleansing lotion or cream, rinse your face thoroughly with warm water and towel dry, then go to bed with a free skin. Even if you have mature, dry skin that needs regular lubricating, you should use it only during the day – ten minutes of absorption is the most a cream can achieve, and anything left on the surface is not needed.

Occasionally, puffiness is genetic. It can be treated by applying eye gels or eye pads which have been soaked in cold eye lotion. (To make the lotion cold, put it in a small, empty pill bottle, and rest it in a basin filled with ice cubes until the lotion is cold.) Ice packs have

> **6** *Puffy eyes are generally caused by leaving creams on the face overnight.* **9**

long been used to reduce swelling from sprains and, provided the eye pads are not left on the eyes too long, this treatment should help.

Cosmetic surgery (see page 114) is the answer if the condition is a longterm one and you have tried all the foregoing suggestions; this solution can have fabulous results.

CELLULITE

Cellulite is the inflammation of the tissues caused by trapped toxic waste due to the lymphatic drainage not activating sufficiently. There are many reasons for this. It could be due to hormonal disturbances caused by pregnancy, the menopause or the contraceptive Pill, or it could be the result of bad circulation and overweight.

When you are overweight, fat deposits cover the lymph nodes, which are 'open-ended' ducts that transport the waste matter into the central lymphatic system, where it is then processed to the kidneys for elimination from the body. The action of muscles is required to push the waste along, and so overweight people suffer in two ways. Firstly, the ducts are blocked with fat, and, secondly, the muscles are usually weak because of lack of exercise. Consequently, a build-up of waste matter is inevitable. The only way to eliminate this is to reduce weight and take up exercise to combat the problem.

A treatment bath of Epsom salts will help to soften the area and draw out some of the waste matter. Pour four cupfuls of commercial Epsom salts (available from chemists) into a hot bath and then soak in the water for at least half an hour. Do not try to wash in the water – just relax. It should cause you to sweat heavily. Afterwards, rest in bed for a further half hour. A loofah rubbed over the region will help improve circulation and thereby increase the cleansing activity. There is no need to use expensive cellulite gels or other such preparations, though they will do you no harm and can soften the skin.

When men reach middle age and their hormone levels change, they also become prone to this condition, but it usually occurs around their midriff and tummy area because this is the part of their anatomy where they lay down the fatty deposits.

Thin women with this condition are usually afflicted if they have bad circulation or low muscle tone.

If hormonal causes have triggered the development of cellulite, then a good result can often be obtained.

With age, it is inevitable that the system of lymphatic drainage will

> ❛ *A good cellulite treatment is an Epsom salts bath, which draws waste matter from the skin.* ❜

get less and less effective. Although keeping your weight down and carrying out a few stretching and toning exercises will help to keep the dimply effect under control and make it less noticeable, the loss of elasticity in the tissues will eventually make cellulite unavoidable.

STRETCH MARKS

Another problem I commonly come across is stretch marks, not only in women who are or have been pregnant but also in overweight people and in teenagers. The marks, which appear on breasts, stomach, hips and thighs, are caused by excessive or rapid weight gain, as in pregnancy or the fast growth that happens during puberty. In other words, the skin has been stretched beyond its natural capacity.

Because the elasticity of skin varies from person to person, some people are more prone to stretch marks than others. Pregnant women of any age can develop them, but there is a greater chance of the marks occurring over the age of about 35, when the dermis is beginning to thin and lose its natural elasticity. There is also a possibility that an excess of corticosteroid hormones in the body could be a contributing factor; these hormones are known to suppress fibre formation in the skin, so that the skin's collagen dries out, reducing its elasticity.

Stretch marks appear initially as fine red lines. Unfortunately, they never disappear entirely, because the damage done to the underlying tissues is permanent. They do, however, fade to a silvery colour, becoming much less noticeable. Some skin clinics carry out laser treatments, but I know of no satisfactory treatment to remove stretch marks. Keeping the skin well lubricated will make it look smoother so that the marks are less apparent.

Various specially formulated creams are available to massage into the skin in order to prevent stretch marks from forming, but any

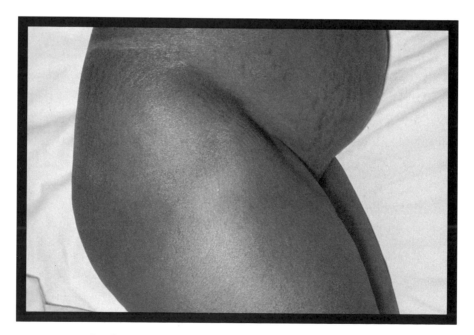

Heredity determines whether a person will be prone to stretch marks.

benefit from them is more likely to be due to the massaging action than to the creams themselves, which cannot penetrate to the dermis where the damage occurs.

PREGNANCY

During pregnancy, the body's raised levels of oestrogen, progesterone and other hormones can alter your complexion. In the first few months, when your body is still adjusting to these new hormone levels, your skin may become more prone to spots. As the pregnancy advances, however, the spots will probably disappear, and a rosy glow will emerge, making your skin look quite radiant. The glow is caused by the dilation of the blood vessels near the skin's surface, due to the increased hormone level. Sometimes, in fact, the enlarged blood vessels may become rather too noticeable, but this effect will recede within about six weeks of the birth.

Stretch marks too may appear during pregnancy – these are covered on pages 97–9.

Skin (and hair) may become oilier, or occasionally drier, and cases of acne often improve or even clear up for good. If you are taking antibiotics for acne, your doctor will probably advise you to stop taking them while you are pregnant.

Nipples, pigmented moles, freckles and birthmarks generally darken, and pigmentation also causes the barely visible line that runs from the breasts to the groin to darken; this will fade within a year of the birth. Sometimes in late pregnancy, hyperpigmentation of the skin develops. Known as chloasma, or the 'mask of pregnancy', it appears as dark patches on the cheeks, upper lip, forehead or neck. The sun can make the patches worse, so if you have developed chloasma stay out of the sun as much as possible, or at least use a sunblock. Do not use a bleaching cream while you are pregnant. The dark patches will fade after pregnancy, but they disappear less easily if they have been exposed to sunlight.

Another problem that can develop during pregnancy as a result of sun exposure is photosensitivity. See page 111 for advice about this.

Bumps and rashes may also develop during pregnancy. Usually due to a change in hormonal levels, they can be very distressing. The lumps look like blind boils (boils caused by bacterial invasion) and can be very painful. It is difficult to deal with the problem because a doctor must look after the welfare of the unborn baby and he/she knows that the problem will right itself after the birth. My suggestion is to use unperfumed cleansing cream and wash the cleanser away with warm water then pat dry. Avoid using too much moisturizer (though if your skin has become very dry, that may be difficult). Apply conditioning cream only to the dry area, leaving the rash and bumpy area alone. Check your diet and discuss with your doctor whether you might need a vitamin and mineral supplement. Try to have a monthly facial – the combination of the relaxation it engenders and the gentle exfoliation from the facial massage can help to clear your skin.

After the birth, the sudden drop in hormone levels, combined with the effects of stress and lack of sleep, may lead not only to severe hair loss but also to the scalp and skin becoming either very oily or very dry. In addition, dandruff, a coarsening of facial hair, spots and blackheads may develop. (These problems are dealt with elsewhere in this book.) Console yourself with the fact that the problems are temporary – your skin and hair *will* eventually return to normal.

THE MENOPAUSE

One of the symptoms of the menopause is extremely dry skin, leading to a more rapid and visible ageing of the complexion. This is caused by the reduced level of oestrogen, the hormone that keeps the skin smooth, moist and resilient. In addition, facial hair often becomes more noticeable during the menopause, but there are methods of dealing with this (see pages 74–7 and 83). The most common symptom is the hot flush, a sudden feeling of heat that spreads up to the face and lasts for several minutes. On fair skin, in particular, this is very noticeable as blushing. It is a distressing sensation and, although it only lasts a few minutes, it feels like an eternity.

Hormone Replacement Therapy (HRT), which replaces the lost hormones until the menopausal symptoms cease, will help enormously with these problems. If, however, you cannot go on HRT, try taking vitamin E and ginseng. There are also vitamin and mineral tablets specifically formulated for women undergoing the menopause.

ILLNESS

Skin reflects a person's state of health and the complexion can easily look 'flat' after an illness. Here is how to perk it up. First, change to a cream cleanser and become fanatical about cleaning your skin gently. Massage the cream into the face and neck, removing it with cotton wool that has been soaked in warm water and then sprinkled with rosewater. Do not use any scrubs or rubs – instead make up a kaolin mask (see page 48), mixing it with full-fat milk rather than water to make a glossy cream. Paint it on to the skin, then put some rosewater

Look after yourself from the inside and it will show on the outside.

eye pads on to the eyes and lie down for ten minutes. Remove the mask with warm water, and finish off with a spray of rosewater. Apply the mask on a weekly basis, and carry out the cream cleaning daily until the skin softens up.

Illness affects hair and nails, too, so treat them to some tender loving care as well. Look after yourself from the inside and it will show on the outside. Vitamin and mineral supplements can make a lot of difference after illness. Consider a change of hair colour – not a radical change but something to give you an instant lift.

CHAPTER FIVE

SUN PROTECTION

P reventing sun damage is the most important thing you can do for your skin. The sun can wreak havoc with it unless you take certain important precautions. Yet, with the plethora of sun creams and lotions available today, and the increasingly technical jargon accompanying them, it is not surprising that many people simply continue with their old bad habits.

ULTRA-VIOLENCE

If you intend to go out in the sunshine, or to use a sunbed, then it is essential that you protect your body from the adverse effects of sunlight. The sun emits two types of ultraviolet rays that reach the earth – which are known as UVA and UVB rays. Originally, it was thought that only the UVB rays caused skin damage, since they are the rays responsible for sunburn.

However, it now appears that, in fact, the UVA rays do more longterm damage than the UVB rays. They penetrate further into the skin, into the dermis, where they cause untold damage which leads to the signs of premature ageing of the skin, and sometimes to skin cancer. The sun emits infra-red rays (radiant heat) too; these are now also thought to be linked with cancer and other forms of skin damage. And today, with the damage to the earth's ozone layer, a greater amount of solar radiation is reaching the earth, making sunbathing even more dangerous.

THE TANNING PROCESS

A suntan is actually the body's response to the threat that the sun poses. Sunlight stimulates the skin to increase its production of the pigment melanin. As the melanin supply increases, it moves up to the surface of the skin, where it acts like a filter to help prevent burning and reduce the penetration of the rays. This process usually takes

> *A suntan is actually the body's response to a threat.*

two or three days. As more and more pigment reaches the surface, the skin gets darker.

Everyone has an inbuilt melanin quota, or maximum amount of melanin that the skin can produce. Those people who have fair skin and/or light eyes cannot usually achieve as dark a tan as someone with naturally darker skin or eyes.

SUN DAMAGE

Continued over-exposure to the sun will eventually make skin thick, dry, leathery and prematurely wrinkled. It can also cause wartlike growths called solar keratoses, which in turn may lead to skin cancer. Whereas this is the result of steady exposure to daylight over a long period of time, another, more deadly type of skin cancer – malignant melanoma (see page 94) – is thought to be related to short, sharp overdoses of sun, such as a severe sunburn occurring during a holiday in a hot climate.

Over-exposure to the sun also has a number of other unpleasant side-effects, including photosensitivity (see page 111), heat rash and heatstroke. Of course, it does also have its benefits, particularly sunlight's recognized ability to relieve stress, and its boosting of immune cell production.

CHOOSING SUNSCREENS

There is such a bewildering choice of sunscreens available now that I'm sure many people decide it's simpler not to bother with one. But a good sunscreen is absolutely vital. Look for a broad-spectrum product, which will provide protection against UVA as well as UVB rays.

Choose a sunscreen with a high SPF (sun protection factor). The higher the number, the greater the level of protection, since the number indicates how much longer it will enable you to stay out in the sun without burning. For instance, if you normally would burn after 15 minutes, a sunscreen with SPF 10 would allow you to stay in the sun for 10 x 15 minutes, or 2½ hours. (This principle does not strictly apply beyond SPF 15; SPF 30, for instance, blocks 98 per cent of the rays, while SPF 15 blocks 95 per cent. Also, the SPF is only a measure of the sunscreen's protection against UVB rays; at present there is no standardized method of indicating UVA protection.) Remember that a high SPF does not give you the licence to stay out in the sun indefinitely: no sunscreen offers complete protection.

The fairer your skin, the more likely you are to burn. People with freckles and people with blonde or red hair and blue or hazel eyes also burn very easily. Furthermore, those who burn easily are at the highest risk of developing skin cancer.

Once you have selected a sunscreen to suit your skin type, you can use the same factor throughout your holiday. There is no need to buy a number of different factors – simply re-apply the high factor less frequently towards the end of your holiday when your skin has tanned. As a general guide, those whose skin burns easily should use a sunscreen with a SPF greater than 10. Those who tan easily but

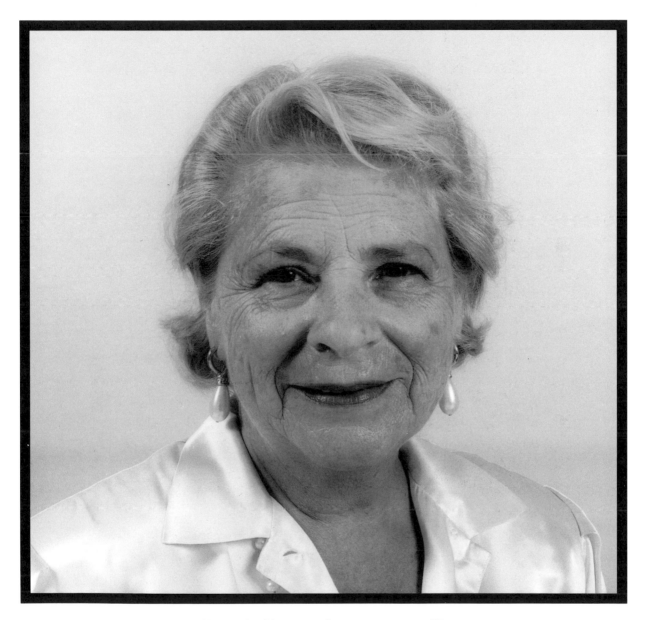

The sun's effect on the skin may not become apparent until later years.

sometimes burn should use SPF 8 or higher. And those who tan easily and rarely burn should use at least SPF 6.

Sunscreens come in many formulations, including creams (especially in the higher SPFs), lotions, oils (in the lower or even zero SPF ranges), sticks (for specific areas such as eyelids, nose, lips), mousses and gels. Total sunblocks reflect all the light rather than filtering out a proportion of it. Some sunscreens are water-resistant, an essential feature if you plan to swim.

SAFER SUNBATHING

Follow these guidelines to make your sunbathing safer. (And remember, you actually need sun protection whenever you are outside, even if you are just walking the dog or gardening. Men are the worst culprits for neglecting their skin, as they think they are too 'manly' to wear sunscreen.)

♦ If you are prone to burning, avoid sunbathing as much as possible.

♦ Wear loose-fitting clothing when walking around in the sun, and a wide-brimmed hat whenever possible.

♦ If you have any skin trouble, pigmentation problems or rashes, you should apply a total sunblock in the sun.

♦ Put your sunscreen on before you go out in the sun, and before you put on your swimsuit, so that every bit of exposed skin will be protected. Re-apply it after swimming, as well as every hour for the first few days of a holiday and then every couple of hours. Sweating, swimming, and towel-drying all wear it away.

♦ Be sure to protect vulnerable or sensitive areas such as the nose, lips, eyelids, cheeks, back of the neck, shoulders, upper chest, nipples, soles and tops of feet, shins and backs of legs and knees.

♦ Avoid sunbathing between the hours of 11am and 3pm, especially at the beginning. This period is when the sun is fiercest. And remember that, as well as the time of day, the time of year and location also affect the intensity of the sun. The effect of sunlight is more intense near the equator (because the angle at which the rays strike the earth is sharper) and at high altitudes (because the thinner atmosphere filters out fewer UVB rays).

♦ Snow and white sand reflect sunlight, so the rays can attack you coming *and* going! Other surfaces also reflect light, which is why you can burn in the shade. You can also burn on a cloudy day.

♦ Avoid falling asleep in the sun unless you are with someone who will wake you up in time. Take your sunbathing in easy stages, and don't overdo it – you may not recognize when you have had enough. Sunburn can appear up to 24 hours after exposure.

♦ Protect your eyes too. The paler they are, the more sensitive they will be in the sun. Avoid exposing your eyes to strong sunlight. Too much sunlight can damage them, so a good pair of sunglasses is essential. (Any white marks can be disguised with a tinted moisturizer or fake tan if necessary.)

CHILDREN IN THE SUN

Dermatologists estimate that about 50 per cent of sun damage occurs before the age of twelve. Skin cancers can appear in children as young as four. Children have thinner skin than adults until they reach adolescence, and tanning mechanisms are not fully developed in young children. Keep babies less than six months old out of direct sunlight, and do not use a sunscreen on babies of this age. Older infants should be protected with light clothing, a wide-brimmed hat and a sunscreen with a high SPF on exposed skin. It is vital that children get into the habit of protecting their skin against the sun.

AFTERSUN TREATMENT

When you come in from the sun, let your body cool down for half an hour or so then have a lukewarm bath or shower.

Hot, dehydrated skin will benefit from an aftersun lotion, which will help to soothe and cool it down, as well as lubricating it. Aftersun products come in a variety of formulations, including mousse and gel, lotion and cream. As well as basic moisturizing or soothing ingredients like aloe vera, jojoba, cocoa butter, witch hazel, camomile, cucumber, avocado oil or sunflower oil, many contain 'extras' such as vitamins A, E or B5 or insect repellents. However, if you are in the habit of using a body lotion, this product is all you need to keep your skin soft and resilient after sunning.

Keeping your skin moisturized will help prevent a tan from peeling, but if you have overdone the sunbathing, the damage is done and peeling is unavoidable.

To treat sunburn, either aspirin or ibuprofen (or paracetamol for people sensitive to those drugs and for children under twelve) will reduce the discomfort. Drinking plenty of fluids is also important. Take cool rather than warm baths or showers, and avoid using soap or bath foam, which would irritate and dry out the skin even more.

A soothing lotion or mousse such as calamine will help relieve soreness and itching. Sunburn creams and sprays with 'caine' in the name, such as benzocaine, contain local anaesthetics to ease the pain, as well as antiseptics to help prevent infection (often a serious side-effect of sunburn). Severe cases of sunburn, in which the skin is blistered and the person is unwell, should be treated by a doctor. Moderate cases will usually subside in about five days – but the damage to underlying tissues is permanent.

SUNBEDS

Sunbeds used to be regarded as the safe way to get a suntan, as they emit mainly UVA rays. However, now that the dangers of UVA rays are known, sunbeds are recognized as being at least as risky as the sun itself, and probably even more so. What really concerns me about sunbed treatments, particularly the 'high-powered' sunbeds, is how the body is signalled to produce melanin so quickly. The skin is bombarded with ultraviolet at such an intensity that a noticeable tan develops after the first half-hour session. Surely there is an interaction with other chemicals in the body and, in consequence, an increased risk of skin cancer occurring.

Anyone who burns easily should avoid sunbeds completely, since they could do untold damage to their skin and, at any rate, will not develop a good tan from a sunbed anymore than they would from the sun. (Only those who tan easily in the sun can get much colour from a sunbed.) Anyone at greater risk of developing skin cancer (those with a family history of malignant melanoma, or with a history of severe

> *What really concerns me about sunbeds is how the body is signalled to produce melanin so quickly. The skin is bombarded with ultraviolet.*

sunburn, particularly in childhood, or with a propensity to freckling) should also avoid it, as should children under the age of sixteen.

I do not recommend the use of sunbeds; but if you are determined to subject your skin to this onslaught, then at least follow these guidelines.

♦ Avoid the high-powered, fast-tanning type of sunbed.

♦ Do not use a sunbed on a regular basis for any length of time, certainly not for more than two courses a year (each of which should be no more than ten sessions).

♦ Only use a sunbed at a salon that supervises clients, has shower facilities and provides protective goggles.

♦ Pregnancy and certain drugs (see page 111) can sometimes sensitize the skin to ultraviolet. If in doubt, do not use the sunbed.

♦ Shower before using it, in order to remove perfume, deodorant and make-up, which can sensitize the skin to ultraviolet.

♦ Wear protective goggles when taking a sunbed treatment, and do not exceed the recommended time (an absolute maximum of 30 minutes).

♦ Remember that you will still need to use a sunscreen with a high SPF when you go out in the sun.

♦ Stop using the sunbed if you develop such side effects as redness, freckling or heat rash (which 50 per cent of users do).

QUESTIONS FROM CLIENTS

I have dark skin, so can I forget about wearing a sunscreen?

The extra melanin in black skin provides excellent protection against the sun, which is why black skin does not develop the signs of ageing as rapidly as white skin. In fact, sun can give black skin a healthy, radiant glow. Nevertheless, black skin will burn if over-exposed, and so will benefit from a sunscreen. The lighter your skin tone, or paler your eyes, the higher the SPF you will need. If you develop any pigmentation problems do not go out in the sun and do consult your doctor.

I often get cold sores after sunbathing. What can I do?

Cold sores can indeed be triggered off by strong sunlight – and they may also appear when your resistance is low. Herpes simplex, as the condition is known, cannot at present be cured; once you have suffered an attack, the virus stays with you for life. It is *very* infectious and can be transmitted by contact with another person's skin. Avoid picking at the sores, wash your hands thoroughly after touching them, and do not share towels. Take particular care to prevent the virus from affecting the eyes – don't rub your eyes after touching the sores, and if you wear contact lenses, never use saliva to wet the lenses. Obviously you should avoid sunbathing, even on a sunbed, if you want to prevent further outbreaks. If you begin to feel that telltale prickling that signals an attack, dab a drop of cold coffee on the site, continuing to apply it until the prickling has stopped. For some reason it seems to help prevent the sore from developing. There are also soothing, antiseptic treatments available at the chemist's.

I've started getting an itchy red rash on my arms after sunbathing.
What could be causing it?

In some people ultraviolet rays penetrating the skin can
cause chemicals stored there to trigger off a reaction. This
may include redness, itchiness or swelling, and blistering,
usually on the neck, shoulders, chest and arms. These
chemicals, or photosensitizers, come from such everyday
substances as perfumes, perfumed soaps and deodorants;
citrus fruits; figs, carrots and celery (if eaten in large
quantities); some fruit juices and low-calorie drinks; as well
as certain tranquillizers, antihistamines, antibiotics,
antidepressants, asthma drugs, painkillers, the Pill or
Retin-A (see page 91). Pregnancy too can have this effect. If
you are prone to photosensitivity, are pregnant or are on
photosensitizing medication, you should avoid the sun
completely, or at least wear a total sunblock.

Are cosmetics containing sun filters any use?

Many make-up and skin-care products now contain
sunscreens. Often, the SPF is quite low, so they do not
provide adequate protection when sunbathing, but they are
useful for day-to-day wear.

I have quite fair skin but I never go abroad for holidays, so I don't really
need to use suncream, do I?

Yes! Obviously a stronger suncreen is necessary in hot countries,
which are nearer the equator and where the sun is consequently
fiercer. But even in relatively cool climates the sun will inflict
permanent damage on your skin – often without any visible
signs at the time – unless you wear a sunscreen.

CHAPTER SIX

COSMETIC SURGERY

If, despite looking after your skin, you are beginning to see a heaviness around the eyes and a sagging jawline, the only real remedy is cosmetic surgery. There have been lots of scare stories connected with this, but you hear less from the thousands of satisfied patients. Consequently, whenever cosmetic surgery is mentioned, there is a shudder of fear. Let's look objectively at the subject.

BASIC CHOICES

The way recommended by most magazines and press articles is to consult your doctor. This is obviously a good suggestion but there are many doctors who do not know one cosmetic surgeon from another and have no yardstick by which to measure one surgeon's technique against another's. Beauticians, however, are in constant touch with the subject. Even if they have not personally had surgery, they see many clients who have and they can assess the work of various surgeons, who tend to specialize in a particular area. Discussing the matter with a beautician can help to take the fear out of the visit to the surgeon, because the beautician is aware of the preparation required and the post-operative effects. She is on hand to listen and advise and even to introduce one client to another so that they can compare notes.

Cosmetic surgery is not for the lady who is unhappy with herself, who hates her own image and would prefer to be someone else. In fact, this person would be disappointed with the results, because all that cosmetic surgery does is to make you look more rested. The heavy lines are gone and the eyes seem wider; necks and jowls lose their sag, and a firmer face emerges. But it is still *your face*.

> **❛ *You will come out of the surgery looking as though you have gone a round with Frank Bruno.* ❜**

Something else to be aware of is the post-operative appearance. You do not come out of surgery without some swelling and bruising, so you will not look great straightaway. In fact, you will look as though you have gone a round with Frank Bruno. Also, there is a loss of feeling in the cheek area at first, though this comes back within a few weeks when the whole face begins to settle down to its new look.

CONSULTATION

When you have selected the surgeon, either through your doctor or through your beautician, make a list of questions you would like answered. Do *not* take a photograph of a celebrity or even one of you at eighteen; these changes cannot be done. Here is a list of some points to discuss with your surgeon:

♦ What type of scarring will there be?

♦ How long will you stay in hospital?

♦ If you are taking any medication, tell the surgeon, for it could have adverse effects, perhaps on the way your blood will clot.

♦ Is the surgery painful?

♦ What is the period of recovery? Are there any post-operative treatments you need to undertake?

♦ Some techniques are now carried out under local anaesthetic.Discuss with the surgeon whether your operation could be carried out in this way.

♦ What are the costs involved? Does it include hospital and anaesthetist's fees?

♦ If you smoke, you should mention this to the surgeon because it may be a factor in your recovery.

The surgeon will also ask you questions. These will enable him to ascertain whether you are physically and psychologically balanced enough to undergo this type of surgery. Surgeons are very aware of some people's unhappiness and distress, and they would not undertake surgery of this nature on someone with a psychological problem.

> **6** *Cosmetic surgery is not for the lady who would prefer to be someone else. In effect, all that it does is make you look more rested.* **9**

Some people go to a consultant for reassurance, with no intention of undergoing surgery. A good surgeon usually accurately assesses this type of person, suggesting they go away and come again in six month's time.

If you are happy with the answers given to you by the surgeon, settle a date for the operation. After that, my advice is to forget about it until a few days before you go into hospital. If you do not, you may lose your nerve. Do not discuss it with your 'best friend'. They have a habit of making you appear vain, or, if that does not work, they try to frighten you with scare stories. (But these tales never happen to anyone they actually know – it is always a vague 'someone'!)

EYE SURGERY

Of the many types of cosmetic surgery available, the most popular and most successful for immediate good looks must surely be the eyes. Blepharoplasty is the term for upper and lower eye surgery. This operation can be carried out by either local or general anaesthetic and is relatively painless. The scarring is minimal and usually is undetectable after a few months. You must expect to have swollen eyes and be bruised initially, however: the shock you may feel if you are not actually expecting this can be severe. But take heart! It does all disappear.

The incision on the top lid is made in the natural crease of the eyelid and is not noticed. The incision at the bottom of the eye is under the lower lashes and is consequently hidden by them. Itching is a problem when recovery is taking place but you will be advised about ice compresses and you can expect to be presentable to the public gaze in about ten days. Eyesight is not affected.

FACELIFTS

The medical name for a facelift is rhytidectomy. Carried out on both men and women, it is usually performed on someone who has a sagging jawline and deep muscle wrinkles. This type of surgery does not take away the fine lines around the eyes and mouth; they can only be removed by chemical peeling or dermabrasion (see page 118).

There is no preferred age for a facelift, but it usually takes place from around the forties upwards. It is not so helpful in old age. A facelift will not change the shape of your face – it will simply make you look rested and give a fresher look to the face. The stay in hospital for this type of surgery is about three days.

A general anaesthetic is preferred but the operation can be done under local anaesthetic. The incisions for the face are made inside the ears; for the neck, which is always included in a facelift, they are made at the back of the head above the hairline. It sounds frightful but it is painless and the incisions heal very quickly.

The worst aspect is the fact that you cannot wash your hair for about six days, although you can clean your hair with warm water three or four days after the surgery.

One of the myths about facelifts is that a skin damaged by over-exposure to the sun and wind cannot be repaired by surgery. In fact, the loose skin can be lifted, but elasticity, once gone, has gone for ever. Also, despite claims to the contrary, lasers, acupuncture and the like cannot take the place of surgical treatment. Should you be in any doubt, please consult your surgeon.

NOSE SURGERY

The reshaping of the nose is known as rhinoplasty. This operating procedure is performed inside the nose and there are no visible scars. If the nostrils are to be made smaller, this will result in small scarring but it will not be noticed when the incisions have healed.

Again, there is very little pain – just discomfort. There will be splints and bandages to contend with, and swelling and bruising are usual. It is a good idea to use a humidifier in your home to prevent the nasal passages from getting too dry. You will be advised not to blow your nose for at least three weeks after your operation and will be asked to clean your nostrils with a cotton wool bud soaked in a solution of warm water and hydrogen peroxide.

You should sleep upright for the first few days after this surgery. As you do not want to put any strain on your face you should not chew heavy food for a while – stick to a light diet. You may not be able to wear eyeglasses for a while after the operation. Once the splints are removed you should be able to wash your hair.

The effect achieved with this operation is extremely rewarding, although it will be many months before your nose will have settled into its new shape.

BREAST SURGERY

Breast reduction is regarded as a major operation and is performed under general anaesthetic. The surgeon will make three incisions: one to reset the nipple (which means a scar in this area), one from the nipple to the base of the breast and a third under the curve of the breast.

Fat and spare tissue are removed and then the breast is re-aligned. There is no pain, only discomfort, and a week away from work is all that is required. Because muscle is not cut, the healing takes place quickly. The scars heal well, and fading around the nipple is such that eventually even this scar will not be visible, as it will merge with the tissue.

Breast augmentation is one of the most requested operations. The traditional method is to have a cut made under the breast and an

> **❛ Breast augmentation is one of the most requested operations. ❜**

implant containing silicone gel inserted. A new technique is to make an incision under the armpit, but this is not always satisfactory because the implant has to be placed very carefully to avoid creating, in effect, another small bosom.

For both types of breast augmentation operation, the post-operative healing is good and the scars fade and merge with the surrounding tissue quite quickly. Again, a week to ten days away from work is required after a hospital stay of one or two nights.

REMOVAL OF SPOT FAT

Removal of spot fat, or liposuction, is a new and important surgical technique. It involves the introduction of enzymes to the area to be treated, and these break down the fat cells into liquid form. The fat is then literally sucked out.

I have seen this used on a thick tummy and under the chin of clients, who now look fantastic. It is also used on heavy thighs and upper arms. It is not recommended by surgeons on people over the age of 50 because the skin has lost a lot of its elasticity.

If this treatment is used on the tummy, a corset must be worn for several weeks after the operation. Bruising and swelling are present for a while. You can expect to look good within about six months.

> *6 I have seen liposuction used on a thick tummy and under the chin of clients, who now look fantastic. 9*

The joy of it is that the fat is gone for ever. Once the fat cells are removed, they cannot replace themselves.

REMOVAL OF SCARS AND TINY LINES

Chemabrasion (chemical peeling) and dermabrasion are two treatments used for the removal of deep acne scarring, chickenpox scars, those dreaded tiny lines around the mouth and the lines that appear due to skin damage following heavy sunning. This type of treatment cannot be undertaken on olive or darker skin because the difference in the new skintone is too marked. But where it can be effected, the results are wonderful.

If you wish to consider this type of surgery, you should discuss it fully with a reputable surgeon affiliated to the British Association of Aesthetic Plastic Surgeons. If done by an unskilled operator, the effect can be disastrous.

Chemabrasion involves painting a chemical on to the skin which literally burns away the top layer of cells to allow the new skin to emerge. The problem with this procedure is that the skin is left white and continues to be white thereafter. A full-face chemical peel should only by undertaken after clinical details have been taken. You should never, never go to a clinic advertising peeling treatments if they do not conform to the medical association regulations. This is because minute amounts of the chemical may be absorbed into the body and can affect the kidneys and liver, and if you have previously had any suggestion of difficulties in these areas the treatment should not be undertaken.

After the chemical solution has been painted on the face, a waterproof adhesive tape is applied leaving only the eyes, lips and nostrils free. There is a burning sensation which can be uncomfortable, or even painful, depending on your pain threshold. This mask is left on for 48 hours.

As in all cosmetic surgery, you should expect itching afterwards, and there is a feeling of tightness which can be intense when the scabs are forming. Plan to allow a period of at least twelve weeks before you show yourself to the public at large. During this time you should stay out of the sun. The advocates of this treatment believe that the smoothness and clearness of the skin after the operation is worth all the tedium of the treatment.

Dermabrasion literally planes, or sands, the skin. Its advocates prefer it because of the control it gives them over the amount of cells that are removed. It is certainly the best method for deep-pitted acne scarring. As with chemabrasion, it is essential to stay out of the sun while your skin is healing afterwards, as the cells will not have had time to form any pigment.

COLLAGEN AND SILICONE INJECTIONS

Collagen injections are now widely used, particularly in the United States, where silicone injections are also being increasingly performed. The purpose is to plump out mouth lines and to lessen heavy nose-to-mouth lines and a deeply furrowed brow. Both methods have many advocates.

Collagen is a compound made from cowhide mixed with distilled water and marketed under the name of Zyderm Collagen. It has three types of thickness and, depending upon the depth required, the surgeon may use a lighter one followed later by the heavier type. You will be asked to have a sensitivity test beforehand to check that you are not allergic to these proteins.

If you suffer from auto-immune diseases such as rheumatoid arthritis, then you would not be given this type of treatment.

The collagen is injected into the area to be treated, which causes the skin to react by allowing normal body fluids to build up in the area. This plumps out the lines. The effect can last several months but, in the end, the collagen will be absorbed into the body, so the injections require regular 'topping up' by the surgeon. This is usually done at three to six month intervals.

Personally, I would only advocate collagen injections if you wanted

> **6 *Collagen injections require "topping up" by the surgeon at three- to six-month intervals.* 9**

a temporary effect for a special occasion, because the effect does not last. One good point, however, is that the American Food and Drug Authority, which is the watchdog of good practice, has passed this animal protein as safe.

Silicone injections involve introducing minute amounts of silicone into a wrinkle, drop by drop. The area is massaged after each injection in order to place the silicone accurately. Silicone is an inert substance and cannot cause an allergic reaction, and it is not cancer-forming. However, once injected into the body, it remains there permanently, so if too much is injected or if it moves out of position, there is no way that the fluid can be retrieved. Because it is not absorbed, there is, in theory, the possibility that it could 'migrate' or move, and form 'pools' of silicone, although U.S. surgeons claim that there is no likelihood of this happening, because it is so finely inserted.

Silicone has not passed the American Food and Drug Authority's safety standards, but it is not illegal to use and is, in fact, a popular treatment in parts of the United States. It is not done in Britain, however.

QUESTIONS FROM CLIENTS

*If I have eye surgery now, will I need to have it done again in the
near future?*

One of the myths you will hear is that you need to have
surgery on your eyes again. This is not so. Eye surgery lasts
for many years – ten to fifteen is not unusual.

*Will I have to change my hairstyle to cover up any scars following
a face lift?*

If you are accustomed to wearing your hair pulled back from
your face, this can still be done when the healing is finished.

*My neck is much more wrinkled than my face. Would chemical
peeling be of any help?*

Neither dermabrasion nor chemabrasion is successful if
applied to a wrinkled neck or hands. The skin in these areas
is not rich enough in oil and hair follicles to be treated
successfully.

*I've been thinking about having liposuction for my large stomach,
but I'm worried about whether there would be scarring.*

With liposuction, the fat is removed in liquid form by vacuum,
rather than being cut away. Only a small incision is made, so
there is no permanent scarring. There is, however, a great deal
of bruising, but this disappears within four weeks or so.

CHAPTER SEVEN

MAKE-UP TECHNIQUES

Make-up has been used over the centuries. Some cultures used it to frighten away evil spirits; for example, the Aborigines in Australia used a white paint mixture to cover themselves, which certainly made them seem frightening. Warriors going into battle used woad and dyes from plants to decorate themselves; the more decorative, the more senior they were, and very elaborate designs evolved. The early Egyptians were renowned for their use of cosmetics. In many cases it was applied to cover defects in skin tone, – which is, of course, equally true to this day. Cosmetics now can enhance and glamorize anyone who develops the correct techniques of application.

The difference between a professional make-up and a bad one is technique. This chapter will help you acquire a professional approach to the application of cosmetics, which will enhance your skin and glamorize your looks.

BASIC TOOLS AND COSMETICS

The essential tools of the trade which you will need are two shaping brushes for eye shadows, one lip brush, one eyeliner brush, two

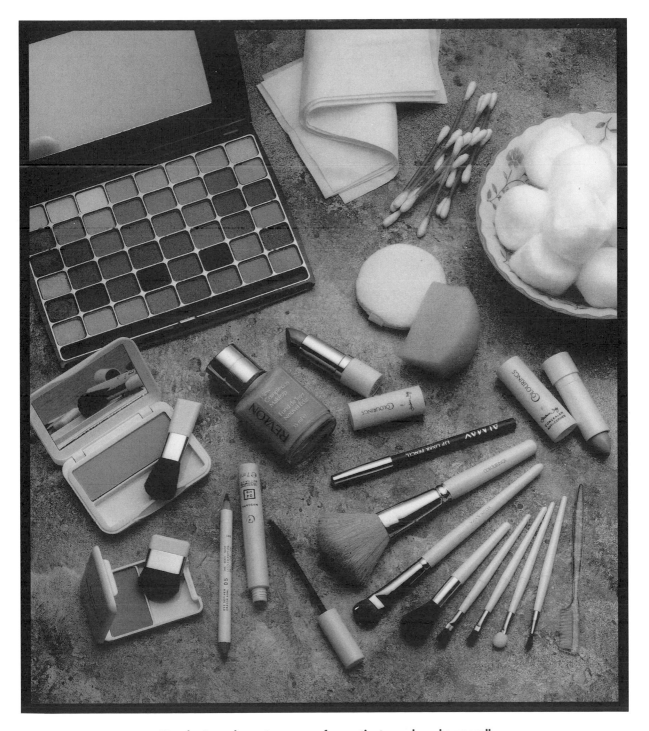

You don't need a vast armoury of cosmetics to apply make-up well.

make-up sponges, cotton wool balls, cotton wool buds, tissues and a good magnifying mirror.

The basic cosmetics you need are a foundation, translucent loose powder, correction stick, a palette of eye colours, blushers (one peach-toned and one pink-toned), and lipsticks to tone with the colours of your clothes.

Colour harmony

Make-up and clothing colours should co-ordinate and harmonize. Here are some examples of colours that work well together.

Outfit Colours	Lipstick	Blusher	Eye Make-up
Greys/black	Clear reds	Nil	Grey/soft silver
Browns/olive/greens	Coral/Peach	Peach	Taupe/bronze
Purple/indigo	Fuchsia	Deep pink	Mauve
Royal blue	Blue reds	Silver pink	Silver/navy

FOUNDATION

Foundation is used to even up skin tones and provide a good base for the rest of your make-up. It is best applied with a barely damp make-up sponge. There are various types of foundation, including creams, blocks, mousses and liquids. If you have high colour or heavy pigmentation you may find a cream best, as it gives the heaviest cover. The block types, which come in compacts and can be used with either a damp or dry sponge, are wonderful if you want to disguise patches of high colour or if you just want a quick touch on the cheeks and nose. They are also good for oily complexions because they tend to be less greasy than other foundations; avoid the oil-free type, however, as they can be too drying. Mousse foundation gives a very light coverage. If in doubt, go for a liquid foundation, as this will give good coverage without being too heavy.

The most important rule to remember for a natural effect is to choose a colour based on your neck tone. Testing colour on the inside

> **6 *If in doubt, choose a liquid foundation, as this will give good coverage without being too heavy.* 9**

of your wrist will give you an idea of how smooth the foundation will look, but it is nowhere near the tone of your face and neck. If you try a small amount of the foundation, and it blends on your neck, it will look very natural when applied to your face.

CONCEALER

A correction stick (or, if you prefer, a concealing cream) is used to camouflage small problem areas such as spots or undereye circles. As with foundation, you should choose one in a shade that matches your neck, though the colours available are much more limited than foundation.

You will get the most natural-looking coverage if you paint the concealer on with a fine brush. Some make-up artists recommend applying concealer underneath foundation, since it is less likely to match the skin as well as the foundation does. Others prefer to apply concealer on top of foundation, as they can use the minimum amount. Whichever sequence you prefer, foundation and concealer must always be followed by powder.

POWDER

Face powder gives your make-up a professional finish and sets your base so that all your make-up lasts longer. Pressed powder is only for touching up your make-up; when applying your base, you must use loose powder. Transclucent powder contains very little pigment and so is ideal for all complexions including dark skins.

APPLYING YOUR BASE

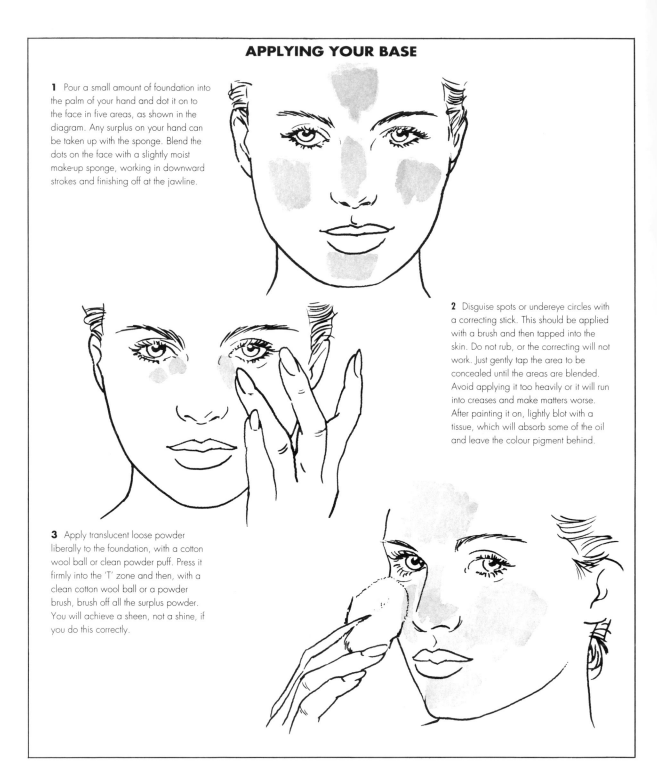

1 Pour a small amount of foundation into the palm of your hand and dot it on to the face in five areas, as shown in the diagram. Any surplus on your hand can be taken up with the sponge. Blend the dots on the face with a slightly moist make-up sponge, working in downward strokes and finishing off at the jawline.

2 Disguise spots or undereye circles with a correcting stick. This should be applied with a brush and then tapped into the skin. Do not rub, or the correcting will not work. Just gently tap the area to be concealed until the areas are blended. Avoid applying it too heavily or it will run into creases and make matters worse. After painting it on, lightly blot with a tissue, which will absorb some of the oil and leave the colour pigment behind.

3 Apply translucent loose powder liberally to the foundation, with a cotton wool ball or clean powder puff. Press it firmly into the 'T' zone and then, with a clean cotton wool ball or a powder brush, brush off all the surplus powder. You will achieve a sheen, not a shine, if you do this correctly.

EYE MAKE-UP

Applied skilfully, eye make-up can emphasize an attractive eye shape and dramatize eye colour. But applied with a heavy hand, it can unbalance the face and detract from the eyes and other features.

Eye shadows

I strongly recommend that you use powder shadows; creams are better left to the true professional.

If you visited a make-up department of a film studio, you would be surprised at the amount of colour that is put on to the eyelid, but the success is in the blending. You must blend, and blend.

> **❛ *I strongly recommend that you use powder shadows; creams are better left to the professional.* ❜**

Study your eye shape. If there is more space by the nose than at the outside edge, then this is where the light colour should be placed, with the darker shade at the outer edge. Reverse this if there is more space at the end of the eye. You can use the sponge applicators that come with the shadows for applying the colours, but you must blend with the brushes for a professional, long-lasting result. Make sure that you blend into the eyelid and not across it, which would only mix the colour. If you have brows that are low down on the eye, it is usually better to line the eye near the lashes and use lots of mascara, rather than using colour on the lids, as that would simply increase the heavy effect and make you look tired.

Eyeliner

You can line with kohl pencils in colours to match your eye, or to tone with what you are wearing, and then blend the line lightly to make it less harsh. Kohl can also be used on the inside of the lower

APPLYING KOHL AND MASCARA

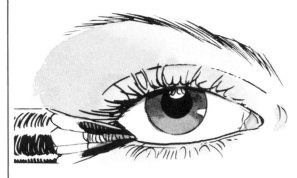

Apply mascara to lashes that have a trace of loose powder on them. Tilt your head slightly and look down your nose into the mirror, so that you can stroke the mascara wand over the underside of the top lashes without poking your eye. On lower lashes the best effect is obtained by using just the tip of the wand and moving the applicator to and fro along the lashes, holding the mirror at eye level and keeping your chin down.

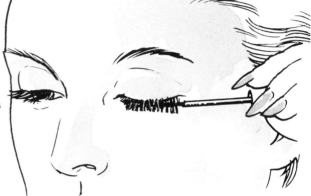

To apply kohl inside the lower lashes, one long stroke will not be effective – you need to use a series of tiny, to-and-fro strokes joining them up as you work along the eye rim. You can also apply kohl to the upper lids along the lash line, to make the eyelashes look more dense. This should be smudged with an applicator to create a softer effect.

lashes to enhance eye colour. Make sure you always use a pencil with the word 'kohl' on it, especially when applying it to the inside of the lower lashes. They come in pencil form and also the newer spiralling crayon type, which are much finer and do not need to be sharpened.

Liquid eyeliner is used to draw a fine line along the eyelid, close to the upper lashes. It needs a very steady hand and, because it cannot be blended, should only be used if you want a strong, definite line.

Eyelashes

Mascara finishes off your eye make-up and adds important definition to your eyes, especially if you cannot use eyeshadows because of heavy eyelids. For the most natural effect, avoid the thick, lash-building types, and apply mascara in thin coats. As you get older, wearing a lot of mascara can be ageing – one or two thin coats will probably be more flattering. Always allow the mascara to dry before applying another coat, combing through the lashes with a stiff eyebrow brush after the mascara has dried in order to separate the lashes. Remove any smudges on your skin with a cotton bud.

FALSE EYELASHES

False eyelashes go in and out of fashion. Provided they are cut to fit, they can be most attractive for special occasions. They usually come in one size only, so they always have to be cut to your own eye shape prior to application. The biggest mistake is applying false lashes that are too wide for the eye or positioning them too high above the natural lashes. Using tweezers and a magnifying mirror will help prevent these problems. Full details are given on page 130.

EYEBROWS

If your eyebrows are really bushy, they must, for appearance, be treated like an overgrown garden. That does not mean to say that you are not allowed thick brows, but they should be shaped. To do this correctly, hold the top of the brow so that the arch becomes obvious and then, with care, tweeze out only the hairs that stand away from the brow. This way, you will avoid taking out hairs from the line itself.

One of the most important points to remember is that the brow should follow on from the line of the nose, so please do not take out hairs from this point as it will unbalance the eyes.

BLUSHER

Blusher finishes the face and makes the eyes look brighter. In addition, it shapes the face and gives a healthy glow. Most cosmetic companies sell a variety of coloured palettes in one container, and I would recommend you go for these so that you can experiment with colour.

Being aware of the shape of your face will help you know where to

APPLYING FALSE LASHES

1 It is a good idea to mascara your own lashes lightly before you begin, as this makes them curl into the false ones, giving the impression of thick lashes.

2 Using a pair of tweezers, hold one up to your eye and place it loosely over your own lashes, with the shortest end towards your nose. You will then see that at least a quarter of the lashes will have to be cut off at the outer end. If the length of the lashes seems too long, you can adjust this too, by cutting into the hair rather than from side to side.

3 To fix the lashes in place, apply the adhesive to a pin, then, holding one set of lashes in the tweezers, run the pin with the adhesive over the top. Using a magnifying mirror for greater visibility, place the lashes above your own and as near to them as possible. Holding your eye taut with your left hand just at the outside of the cheekbone will make this easier, as it elongates the eyelid, so that you can see the line of the lashes.

4 Push one side into place first – usually the side nearest to the nose – and then release the tweezers, pick up the outer part of the lashes and place it in position at the outer corner of the eye. Now press the back of the tweezers along the rim of the false eyelashes to keep them in place.

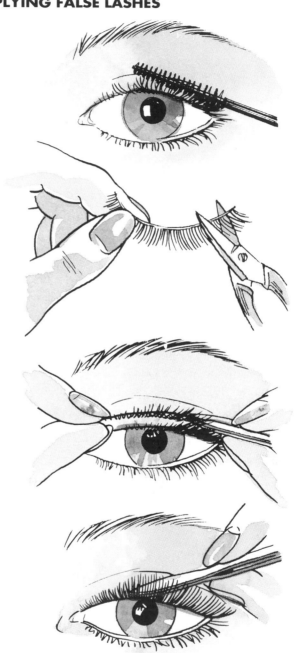

apply blusher to enhance your face rather than detract from it. For example, applying blusher towards the centre of a heart-shaped face would just make it look smaller, while applying blusher towards the temples of a long face would elongate it further. To assess the shape of your face and see where to apply blusher, pull your hair back into a hair band, and study the diagrams on page 132.

LIPSTICK

Lipstick is the final stage in make-up application. Lips vary from one person to another, and if yours are not well-formed or are too thin, you would be well-advised to use only a lip pencil and a little pinky-brown gloss to fill in. This is also advisable for heavy lips.

Always use a lip pencil to outline (you can smooth it out if you wish) and then fill in the lips with a different colour. The best way to use the pencil is to work towards the middle, which gives you more control over your hand.

If your lipstick 'bleeds' into the skin surrounding your lips, you will need to use a pencil first before applying the colour, then blot with a tissue and apply a little powder to the area.

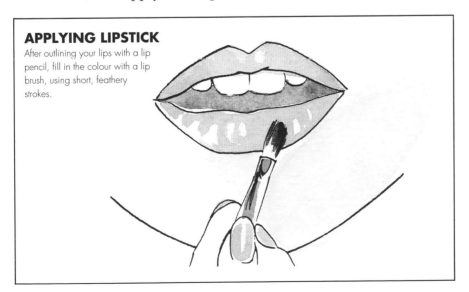

APPLYING LIPSTICK
After outlining your lips with a lip pencil, fill in the colour with a lip brush, using short, feathery strokes.

FACE SHAPES

The drawings show the most flattering positions for blusher in respect of each face shape.

You have a long face if the main part of the face is the middle section with the forehead and chin being equal.

A round face resembles a full moon and usually looks young, even in middle age.

Women with a square face can change their looks quite easily, as cosmetics can create many illusions. You have a square face if you have a large, wide forehead and strong jawline.

Oval faces are rare and are usually considered the most beautiful. The forehead is usually narrow and the chin is pointed while the eyes are large and the nose aquiline.

A heart-shaped face is nearly oval but tends to be small; the chin comes to a point. This shape is very rarely seen on a tall person; it usually is found on a petite person.

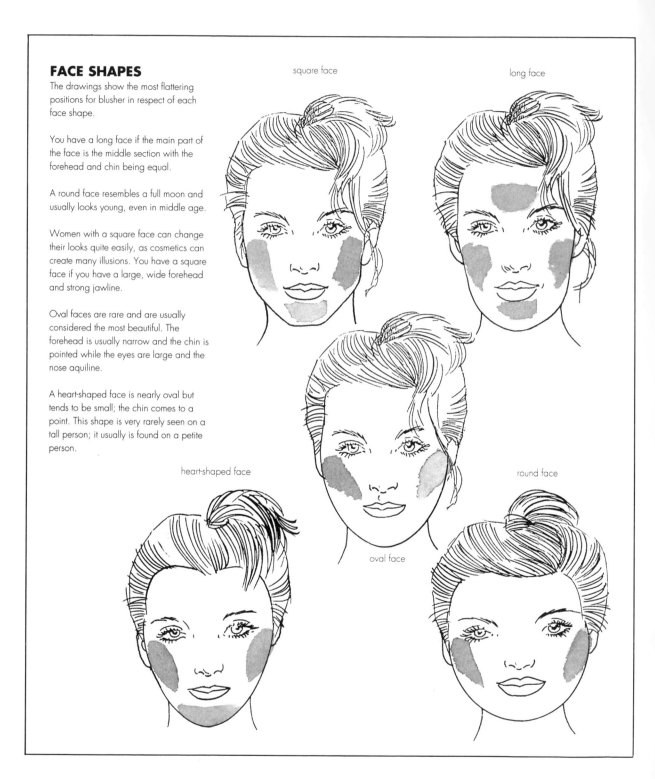

square face

long face

heart-shaped face

oval face

round face

QUESTIONS FROM CLIENTS

My eyelashes are so pale that I have to wear mascara all the time, which is a particular nuisance because I do a lot of sport. Do you recommend having them dyed?

Yes, you could consider having them dyed by a beautician, which will appear to give more depth to the eyes. When hair and skin are both fair, the eyes tend to 'fall back' into the skin, and a little 'pulling forward' with colour creates a more dramatic effect.

Is a correction stick better than a concealing cream?

A correction stick, because of its method of manufacture, will have more pigment in it than a cream, and will therefore provide more coverage. However, even though a correction stick is designed to be dabbed straight on to the skin, it should in fact always be applied with a brush, rather than directly on to the skin, in order to avoid a possible bacterial infection. Using a brush will also make the concealer less noticeable. Concealing cream, too, should be applied with a brush for the same reasons.

Do I have to stop wearing make-up because of my acne?

I am often asked by young girls whether they can wear make-up on skin with acne. I personally feel that as long as it is removed carefully (see pages 32 and 43), you can wear it, as make-up can give you self-confidence when you are feeling desperate. If possible, choose one of the less oily (but not totally oil-free) compact foundations.

CHAPTER EIGHT

THE TOTAL PERSON

A chieving a perfect skin cannot be done overnight. Nor can it be obtained by trying this or that cream or treatment. A beautiful complexion requires an understanding of yourself – knowing what is good for your body and then having the self-discipline to carry out the routine. It does not really matter what goes into a cream: there is no miracle that will make you beautiful. Beauty comes from your own attitude towards yourself.

MAKING THE MOST OF YOURSELF

If you do not like yourself, you will always be seeking to be someone else, which of course leads to failure. It means you will not be making the the most of your own life. We are given wonderful gifts, some of which lie hidden and have to be brought out, while others – such as a good bone structure, wide open eyes, perfect proportions – are more easily recognized.

Each one of our role models has developed her own individual style, which may have taken years to perfect. You can do the same with your own style, taking one day at a time. For example, you may have always loved bright colours but have not dared to wear them because you considered yourself too old, too insecure or simply too price-conscious. Go ahead – develop your new you; you have nothing to lose. Why not change your hair? It can transform your appearance instantly. Ask questions at your hairdresser's to discover just what style would suit you best. Don't limit yourself to what seems trendy or the styles your friends are wearing – the prevailing fashions may not suit you at all. It is *you* we are concerned with.

SKIN SENSE

Skin that has been neglected for years will appear dull and lifeless. But if you begin, as suggested earlier, to take care of your skin by a good, gentle cleansing and conditioning routine, it will begin to show results quickly. It need not take much of your time. Nor does it have to be costly. If you are really serious about this – and I assume you are because you are reading this book – do not be misled by media hype into using too many creams. It really is not necessary. Don't be afraid to look on a supermarket shelf if this makes it easier for you. The packaging may not be glamorous, but the products themselves are of a good and reliable manufacture.

Remember to use sun protection if you are going into the sun or even gardening or walking your dog. Use body lotion all over. You do not need one lotion for the face and a separate one for the body, so choose your favourite. The important thing is to get into the habit of using it regularly and often.

USING COLOUR

As well as your hair and skin, tackle your use of colour – in make-up, and in clothes. Colour can give instant uplift. Perhaps you have stopped using make-up, or maybe your wardrobe is full of neutrals and dull colours. Try holding up various bright colours to your face to see how they can 'lift' your looks, as well as boosting your morale.

There is no point in wearing 'safe' colours – a new image calls for a bold new mental approach.

Colour can give you a more positive outlook. It can transform a dull, drab appearance and uplift your spirits. Yet so many women one sees walking along the street would not be given a second glance. It is not so much a matter of having the money as of having the imagination to incorporate in a wardrobe zingy colours – colours that are bright and alive and that enhance the complexion.

Wearing a colour because it is serviceable is not a good enough recommendation. It can make you depressed and create a negative response in others. If, when looking through your wardrobe, you feel

> **6** *Wearing a colour simply because it is serviceable is not good enough.* **9**

that you have fallen into this trap, stop and consider how you can improve what you already have. Small changes can have a big impact. You might swap the buttons to more exciting ones; add a bright bow; change the collar to bring lightness and brightness to the face.

There are some people who, because they feel self-conscious, do not wear more than one colour – usually either grey, navy blue or black – and variations on that colour. Although it looks neat and tidy (and some have a flair for adding light and dark), somehow it fails to lift them and they end up looking very ordinary.

COLOUR COMBINATIONS

Though people sometimes need a little encouragement, choosing colours can be fun. To get a firsthand insight into colour, try painting your own colour wheel. First, draw a circle and divide it into twelve segments, like pieces of a pie. Now fill in the three primary colours – red, yellow and blue – spacing them equally around the circle.

Mix each pair of neighbouring primary colours together in equal proportions to create the three secondary colours – orange (from red and yellow), violet (from blue and red) and green (from yellow and blue). Position these between the primary colours from which they were made, in other words, directly opposite the primary colour that was not involved in the making of that colour.

Finally, combine pairs of neighbouring primary and secondary colours in equal proportions to form the six tertiary colours (blue-green, red-orange, etc), and paint them into the remaining segments between the colours from which they were made.

Now study the colour wheel for ideas on colour combinations. Colours near each other on the wheel – known as 'toning' colours – look good together and create a harmonious overall effect. Colours opposite each other on the wheel, known as complementary colours, create more striking combinations. When used together, they produce the greatest contrast and seem to bring out the best in each other. Red/green, blue/orange, and yellow/violet are three examples of complementary colour combinations.

'Tints', or 'pastels', are created by adding white to the colours on the colour wheel; most of these are harmonious together. 'Shades' are made by adding black to the colours of the wheel. 'Monochromatic' colour combinations utilize tints and shades from the same colour family – for example, pale turquoise and dark blue-green.

> **6** *There are people who, because they feel self-conscious, usually wear only grey, navy or black. Although it looks neat and tidy, somehow they end up looking very ordinary.* **9**

'Cool' colours are those with blue tones in them, and 'warm' colours are those with yellow or gold in them. 'Neutral' colours are black, white, off-white, beige, browns and greys.

You need to be young, confident and extrovert to wear vividly contrasting colours, or clashing colours like scarlet with fuchsia, or acid yellow with marigold. Generally, it's safer to begin with a toning or monochromatic colour scheme, and add perhaps one small item of a contrasting colour: a large, bright yellow silk rose on a navy jacket with an ice-blue blouse, for example. By the same token, a neutral-coloured outfit can be made much more interesting by spicing it up with a more vibrantly coloured accessory or two – for instance, a touch of rose pink with brown, or a hint of purple with grey.

ENHANCING YOUR SKINTONE

It is important to take your skintone into account when selecting colour. For example, purple or red does not suit people with a highly coloured complexion which is due to capillary damage or red, rosy

> *Anyone with high colouring or a creamy, peachy or olive skin should avoid wearing black and white. They look best on translucent skin with a "blue" note.*

cheeks, as they would only be made to appear more red than they are. It is not a good idea to wear black or pure white with this skintone either; oyster, cool beige and soft, creamy tones are more flattering.

Skin with a cream to olive tone should also avoid black and white. Warm autumnal colours such as orange-reds, yellow-golds, dark chocolate brown and warm beiges will be the most flattering. Lime greens and any colour with a yellow or gold base will bring out the life in this skintone.

Skin with a 'blue' note usually looks good in black and vivid colours such as emerald green or shocking pink. It does not look good in beige or caramel. Translucent, delicate skin fits into this category.

Skin with a peachy tone is enhanced by warm colours but not by white or black. Ivory, camel, peach, yellow-green, bright coral, orange-red, clear aqua blue and light true blue are colours that will bring out the best in this skintone.

COLOUR PLANNING

Using hair or eye colour as the basis for colour planning is not always successful because many women have their hair treated with colour rinses. These change with washing and exposure to sun, chlorine and pollutants, and their reflection can alter the apparent skintone. By working with the actual tone of the skin, the effects of colour are truer, livelier and more stimulating.

Why not begin right now? Examine your wardrobe and throw out anything that you have not worn for a year or more or which you have never really liked.

If you wish to find out more about the fascinating subject of colour, you might like to have your skintone analyzed by a colour consultant who will come to your home and go through your wardrobe with you. They will advise you on what to retain and talk to you about styles and colours that will suit you best.

A TRIM FIGURE

When it comes to taking stock of your weight and figure, bear in mind that you cannot change your skeleton frame. But what you can do is keep your figure trim and firm up your muscles. Although muscles lose some of their firmness with age, exercise will help to prevent the sag and droop that come with total neglect.

It is a great mistake to let the current craze for slimness and food faddism prevent you from enjoying the lifestyle that suits you. Happiness is vital and an important factor in beauty, for it balances the body's rhythms. This is something I feel very strongly about. I have seen anorexic women who have virtually destroyed their lives by trying to be someone else – imagining they are not worth anything and trying to imitate their idol of screen or pop.

Losing weight is not easy, particularly after the age of about forty, but it can be done with slow, gentle determination. Regular exercise will help you lose weight, not only by burning off additional calories but also by boosting your metabolism so that your body uses up

> **6** *Beauty comes from your own attitude towards yourself.* **9**

more calories all the time, even when you are not exercising. A thirty-minute session of reasonably vigorous exercise – such as brisk walking or swimming – three times a week is enough to achieve this effect. As regards dieting, do not skip meals, but reduce all you eat by half (cutting down on fats and sugars, not on vegetables). Avoid alcohol except on very special occasions. Do not set yourself goals that are impossible to obtain – by taking a day at a time you are more likely to achieve your target of a new and revitalized you, *and* to remain there. As I've said before, it all depends ultimately on your attitude towards yourself.

POSITIVE THINKING

When the inevitable 'off days' occur, do not think you have failed. Positive thinking takes time to develop but, once again, the way to achieve it is one day at a time. When I was at my lowest ebb, looking after a mother with Alzheimer's disease and a husband who had had a stroke, and running two businesses at the same time, I used to drive to work at 6.30am singing at the top of my voice 'one day at a time, sweet Jesus', to the surprise of my dog sitting in the passenger seat. It worked. It made me laugh, and that helped set the tone for the day!

So come on. Give it a chance! Let's see happy, healthy, glowing women walking along our High Streets.

INDEX

ACKNOWLEDGEMENTS

I would like to thank the following for their kindness and help in the writing of this book.
Without them I would not have succeeded in doing it.

Judy Woodham, who has so generously given of her time in the typing of the manuscript

Dr Stephen Wright, for his help on the technical aspects of skin care

Mr John Bowen, for his unstinting help and advice on cosmetic surgery techniques

Mr David Stern, my cosmetic chemist, for his support through the years and his advice on
product development

Darley Anderson, literary agent, and Gail Rebuck, Amelia Thorpe and all at Ebury Press
for their encouragement and professionalism.